Psychoanalytic Readings of Hawthorne's Romances

Offering innovative, psychoanalytic readings of Nathaniel Hawthorne's mature novels, this volume expertly applies Freudian theory to present new insights into the psychology of Hawthorne's characters and their fates.

By critically examining scenes in which protagonists confront past traumas, Diamond underscores the transformative potential which Hawthorne attributes to confrontations with the unconscious. Psychoanalytic narrative technique is used to illuminate psychological crises of the protagonists in *The Scarlet Letter*, *The House of the Seven Gables*, *The Blithedale Romance*, and *The Marble Faun*, showing the transformations they undergo to be central to our understanding of the trajectory and resolution of Hawthorne's romances.

The text will benefit researchers, academics, and educators with an interest in applied psychoanalysis, psychoanalytic technique, and Freud in particular. Since its conclusions challenge many currently held critical views, this volume is especially relevant to those interested in interdisciplinary literary studies, Hawthorne studies, 19th century literature and romanticism.

David B. Diamond is a psychoanalyst and psychiatrist in clinical practice. He was formerly Assistant Professor of Psychiatry at Harvard Medical School and served as Director of Outpatient Psychiatry at Brigham and Women's Hospital, Boston, USA.

Psychoanalytic Explorations Series

Books in this series:

The Heart of Man's Destiny
Lacanian psychoanalysis and early Reformation thought
Herman Westerink

Wish-fulfilment in Philosophy and Psychoanalysis
The tyranny of desire
Tamas Pataki

Environmental Melancholia
Psychoanalytic dimensions of engagement
Renee Lertzman

Psychoanalytic Treatment in Adults
A longitudinal study of change
Marian Cogan and John H. Porcerelli

The Unconscious
A bridge between psychoanalysis and cognitive neuroscience
Edited by Mark Solms and Marianne Leuzinger-Bohleber

Psychoanalytic Studies of the Work of Adam Smith
Towards a Theory of Moral Development and Social Relations
Şule Özler and Paul Gabrinetti

Neuroscience, Psychotherapy, and Clinical Pragmatism
Reflective Practice and Therapeutic Action
William Borden

Psychoanalytic Readings of Hawthorne's Romances
Narratives of Unconscious Crisis and Transformation
David B. Diamond

Psychoanalytic Readings of Hawthorne's Romances

Narratives of Unconscious Crisis and Transformation

David B. Diamond

Routledge
Taylor & Francis Group
NEW YORK AND LONDON

First published 2022
by Routledge
605 Third Avenue, New York, NY 10158

and by Routledge
2 Park Square, Milton Park, Abingdon, Oxon, OX14 4RN

Routledge is an imprint of the Taylor & Francis Group, an informa business

Library of Congress Cataloging-in-Publication Data
Names: Diamond, David B., author.
Title: Psychoanalytic readings of Hawthorne's romances: narratives of unconscious crisis and transformation / David B. Diamond.
Description: New York, NY: Routledge, 2021. | Series: Psychoanalytic explorations | Includes bibliographical references and index.
Identifiers: LCCN 2021002082 | ISBN 9780367759094 (hardback) | ISBN 9781003164531 (ebook)
Subjects: LCSH: Hawthorne, Nathaniel, 1804–1864—Criticism and interpretation. | Psychoanalysis and literature. | Psychology in literature.
Classification: LCC PS1892.P74 D53 2021 | DDC 813/.3—dc23
LC record available at https://lccn.loc.gov/2021002082

ISBN: 9780367759094 (hbk)
ISBN: 9780367759100 (pbk)
ISBN: 9781003164531 (ebk)

Typeset in Galliard
by KnowledgeWorks Global Ltd.

To David Kuhn

Contents

Acknowledgments

This book began as a draft of an essay about what I referred to as “the “transformations of Arthur Dimmesdale” in *The Scarlet Letter*. As a psychoanalyst, I was drawn into the vivid psychological world of Hawthorne’s characters and especially to the relentless torments of the guilty minister who finally found release in a long-avoided confession. I applied a psychoanalytic narrative method to derive a fresh understanding of the crisis that brought him to this unanticipated end.

I was extremely fortunate to have David Kuhn, a cherished friend, read the draft. David is an extraordinary poet and literary scholar whose knowledge of literature is encyclopedic and whose literary insights are virtually infallible. Therefore, it took my breath away when he saw great promise in the work; his comment, “after your essay *The Scarlet Letter* will not be read the same,” jolted me into a realization that I indeed had something valuable to contribute to Hawthorne scholarship. Without his confidence in me, at that juncture and at many points later, I would never have had the courage to pursue a series of interpretations of Hawthorne’s romances which also involved a complex journey from psychoanalyst to literary critic. David was my mentor and guide the entire way. He promptly and meticulously read and edited all the analyses as they were being written; his comments inspired me toward more precise formulation and concise expression. It is out of a deep sense of loving gratitude and appreciation for our friendship that I dedicate this book to him.

Chapter Two is the end-product of that initial draft on Dimmesdale and was published in *American Imago*, vol.75, no.4 (2018). The article version of Chapter Four appeared in *Nathaniel Hawthorne Review*, vol. 45, no.1 (2019). *Nathaniel Hawthorne Review* also published Chapter Three in vol. 46, no. 1 (2020). I appreciate having been given permission to reprint the articles in this volume by the Johns Hopkins University Press and Penn State University Press.

It was a pleasure to work with Routledge’s outstanding and congenial editorial team, Elsbeth Wright, Editor—Education, Psychology and Mental Health Research and AnnaMary Goodall, Editorial Assistant. I wish to thank Allison R. Shely who edited and formatted the entire manuscript with intelligence and precision.

I am indebted to my friend, Joel Schultz, for his sustaining interest in the Hawthorne project and for having read and perceptively commented on, in bright red ink, each chapter. His own outstanding Shakespeare scholarship was a model of intellectual integrity and rigor. Wendy Kuhn thoughtfully read drafts of the chapters and offered many important insights. I benefited from Frederick Newberry's years of experience as a Hawthorne scholar and editor. Benjamin Ravid provided counsel and support when I needed it most. Mimosa Stephenson showed great generosity of spirit in reading each and every chapter and superbly editing them. She had faith in the scholarly value of the endeavor and repeatedly encouraged me to collect the essays into a single volume. In many ways she is the guardian angel of this book.

Jonathan F. Borus, Eli L. Diamond, Sharlya Gold, James Kaufman, and David N. Levine have my sincere appreciation for their valuable suggestions regarding various chapters in the book.

1 Introduction

From Tale to Psychological Romance: *The Scarlet Letter*

It is no secret that Nathaniel Hawthorne is a pre-eminently psychological writer. His tales and sketches, the product of the first fifteen or so years of writing were, in Henry James' informed estimation (1879), "glimpses of a great field, of the whole deep mystery of man's soul and conscience" which showed that Hawthorne "cared for the deeper psychology" (p. 65). James was of course correct: Hawthorne was always "a regular dweller in the psychological realm" (p. 65); however, the brevity of his early pieces and undoubtedly his youth did not allow for the complex psychological portrayal and development which are central to his four longer romances. In "Endicott and the Red Cross" (Hawthorne, 1974, Vol. 9) there is mention of "a young woman, with no mean share of beauty, whose doom it was to wear the letter A on the breast of her gown" (p. 435); sixteen years later, this young woman bursts upon the opening scene of *The Scarlet Letter* with an unanticipated vitality of psychological specificity that would determine a literary destiny Harold Bloom (2004) assigned to her: "of all the principal female characters in our national literature, Hester Prynne is clearly the central figure" (p. 4). In the first encounter with this figure, the reader finds that Hester, drawn forward on the threshold of the prison door by the town-beadle, "repelled him, by an action marked with natural dignity and force of character and stepped into the open air, as if by her own free-will. When the young woman—the mother of the child—stood fully revealed before the crowd, it seemed to be her first impulse to clasp the infant closely to her bosom, not so much by an impulse of motherly affection, as that she might thereby conceal a certain token of her shame, which was wrought or fastened into her dress. In a moment, however, wisely judging that one token of her shame would but poorly serve to hide another, she took the baby on her arm, and, with a burning blush, and yet a haughty smile, and a glance that would not be abashed, looked around at her townspeople and neighbors" (Hawthorne, 1962, Vol. 1, pp. 52–53). Hester's dignity, independence, defiance, and canny reckoning with a situation overwhelmingly set against her speaks volumes about her psychology, and does so in a few sentences in which she does not utter a word.

Hawthorne then penetrates beneath his heroine's public attitude of strength to reveal her vulnerability: "she need shriek out with the full power of her lungs, and cast herself from the scaffold down upon the ground, or else go mad at once" (p. 57).

Having gathered experience and confidence, Hawthorne had made a transition from what Robert Milder (2014) calls the "shadowy universals" of the tales and sketches to a truer "explanatory power" of psychological romance in which the writer "was led more deeply than ever before into the minds of his characters...he explored their feelings, motives, impulses and layers of rationalization and denial, along with the historical forces acting upon and within them" (pp. 112–113). Indeed, the "truth of the human heart" which Hawthorne (1962) valorizes in the Preface to *The House of the Seven Gables,* finds expression in the representations of the deepest workings of his characters' psyches. Word for word, paragraph for paragraph, chapter after chapter, there is scarcely a serious work of literature that devotes itself more singularly to the inner life and its conflicts than *The Scarlet Letter.* The small, claustrophobic Puritan colony, with its stark rules of conduct and abundant opportunities for the exercise of voyeuristic zeal, provides a narrow, shallow and brilliantly lit stage against which the inner lives of the intensely entangled, conflicted, and tormented characters are played out. Their secrets, always under pressure of exposure, set them apart from their community, from each other, and from their own selves. They variously suffer severe anxiety, dissociation, depression, obsession, compulsion, and hallucination. Under the burden of psychic strain, each character is prone to forms of psychological deterioration. Hester, Dimmesdale, and Chillingworth are caught in a psychological labyrinth from which there appears to be no exit, and is best described by Hester as "wandering together in this gloomy maze of evil, and stumbling, at every step, over the guilt wherewith we have strewn our path" (Hawthorne, 1962, Vol. 1, p. 174). These characters typify the judgment of *The House of the Seven Gables*: "For, what other dungeon is so dark as one's own heart! What jailer so inexorable as one's self!" (Hawthorne, 1962, Vol. 2, p. 169).

In addition to its pervasive psychological preoccupation, *The Scarlet Letter* is written in what will become, a half century later, the language of psychoanalysis. The pronounced influence of the unconscious on the characters, their inner fantasies and their conflicts, which comprise so much of the substance of the romance, are all solidly within the Freudian ken. Or put more accurately, psychoanalysis will eventually borrow the language of the psyche first inscribed by Hawthorne.

Hawthorne, Freud, and the Haunted Mind

Although *The Scarlet Letter* marks a quantum maturation in his fiction, there is a remarkable consistency in the broad psychological framework Hawthorne employs throughout his writings. The prototype for the system of psychology which informs *The Scarlet Letter* and the three subsequent romances was put forth with succinctness and force in his early sketch, "The Haunted Mind" (1962), which is entirely devoted to the activities of the mind. It will be useful to describe this work in some detail since it constitutes a distillation of what was and what was to be Hawthorne's psychological schema.

The narrator awakens after midnight on a cold winter night. He describes his mind being in "an intermediate space where the business of life does not intrude; where the passing moment lingers and becomes truly the present" (Hawthorne, 1974, Vol. 9, p. 305). In this state, the mind is a more passive recipient of "Passion and Feeling" which are experienced viscerally or "may assume bodily shape, and things of the mind become dim spectres to the eye" (p. 306). We can reword this mental state in the language of psychoanalysis as follows: between sleep and wakefulness the ego's defensive operations slacken and the psyche is more receptive to unconscious contents which are guided by a primary process of emotional and non-logical association. This is, of course, the paradigm of psychoanalytic free-association.

It is in this freely associative zone, where the reality-driven concerns of the *ego* do not hold sway, "Passion and Feeling," which are expressions of the *id* meet the opposing force of the *superego*. It is important to note, too, how this conflict of desire and conscience is condensed, in Hawthorne's imagination, into visual, personified images. In his mind's eye, in an association to a dead man in a coffin, the narrator "sees" a stern figure "with a brow of wrinkles, a look and gesture of iron authority; there is no name for him unless it be Fatality, an emblem of the evil influence that rules your fortunes; a demon to whom you subjected yourself by some error at the outset of life, and were bound his slave forever, by once obeying him. See! those fiendish lineaments graven on the darkness, the writhed lips of scorn, the mockery of that living eye, the pointed figure touching the sore place in your heart! Do you remember an act of enormous folly, at which you would blush, even in the remotest cavern of the earth? Then recognize your Shame" (p. 307). In this mental zone, the past, with its associated deep feelings, haunts the present in the form of visualized, quasi-allegorical figures of Sorrow, Hope, Disappointment, Iron Fatality, and Shame. F.O. Matthiessen (1941) remarks that "the figures may seem no more than traits out of one of Spenser's processional masques, but they are the same traits that dominate all Hawthorne's work" (p. 232). Matthiessen's observation underscores that in these figures Hawthorne's psychology and proclivity toward allegory intersect. As I will amplify in Chapter Two on *The Scarlet Letter*, we can now speak accurately of Arthur Dimmesdale's haunted mind as there is a striking resemblance to the psychic representation of the narrator in the "The Haunted Mind" with that which Dimmesdale sees in a looking glass during one of his midnight vigils: "now it was a herd of diabolical shapes, that grinned and mocked at the pale minister, and beckoned him away with them; now a group of shining angels, who flew up heavily as sorrow laden…now came the dead friends of his youth" (Hawthorne, 1962, Vol. 1, p. 145). In his 1835 "The Haunted

Mind" sketch, Hawthorne was putting forth the template for the dynamics of Arthur Dimmesdale's haunted mind of 1850.

Magisterially, the narrator of "The Haunted Mind" concludes: *"In the depth of every heart there is a tomb and a dungeon, though the lights, the music and the revelry above may cause us to forget their existence, and the buried ones or prisoners whom they hide. But sometimes, and oftenest at midnight, those dark receptacles are flung wide open"* (p. 306, emphasis added). Hawthorne, anticipating Freud, avers that, under certain conditions, primitive and powerful unconscious contents can flood the conscious mind and produce far-reaching disruption of psychic functioning. In this broad statement Hawthorne generalizes about the very nature of the human psyche. It is this comprehension that brings Freud's system closest to Hawthorne's vision. As I will describe, such eruptions of the unconscious become the context for Hawthorne's protagonists' crucial psychological transformations.

In "The Haunted Mind" Hawthorne also drafts the broad outline of what would be central aspects of the Freudian topographic system set forth in *The Ego and the Id*: the division of the psychic territory of the *id*, and *superego*, and the mediating function of the *ego*; the omnipresent unconscious mind which is the locus of affect-laden memories that are always pushing toward consciousness; the permeable interface between the unconscious and conscious mind and the conditions that govern the dynamic flow between them. Thus, a study of Hawthorne's protagonists from a psychoanalytic point of view is totally prefigured by and congenial to Hawthorne.

When Those Dark Receptacles Are Flung Wide: Psychological Transformations within Narrative Gaps

It is my contention, and the chapters of the book set out to demonstrate, that in each of Hawthorne's romances there is a particular scene of great moment in which the "dark receptacles" of a protagonist's haunted mind "are flung wide open" and he or she will urgently need to contend with "the buried ones and prisoners who hide there." This confrontation with the unconscious is the site of a transformation which lies near each romance's psychological, moral, and spiritual core. In addition, the figure of Death, the great teacher in all of Hawthorne's romances, participates as inciting agent in each of these scenes.[1] This is a singular assertion and one that seems reductionistic in a way in which psychoanalysts are often justifiably accused of espousing. However, it is a conclusion at which I arrived post-hoc, that is, after sequentially analyzing the psychology of the protagonists in each romance, a process which took several years. Even after several careful readings of these works, I had not appreciated this pattern which only became discernable after dedicated close psychological readings. In essence, I found what I was not looking for. Because these findings were so consistent, I sensed that I had arrived at a fresh comprehension of the how Hawthorne puts to use his understanding of psychology to organize and propel his romances. It is this comprehension that I would like to share with the reader; individual essays on each of the romances thus morphed into a book. Because of the sequential evolution of this work, a rationale for the psychoanalytic narrative method that I employ is reiterated, with some variation, at the beginning of each chapter. In an attempt to represent as a virtue what is undoubtedly a flaw, I quote a prescription offered in a book which inspired Hawthorne, Bunyan's *Pilgrim's Progress*: "every tub on its own bottom."

What follows summarizes the scenes which will be analyzed at length in each chapter. In *The Scarlet Letter*, the receptacles of Arthur Dimmesdale's haunted mind are flung open as he, in desperation, is lured into agreeing to flee to England with Hester where they would essentially adopt a life of adultery. On his return townward after the encounter, he experiences the full force of hitherto repressed erotic and destructive impulses which sets the context for a profound psychological reckoning; in the solitude of his study, his ego retakes possession of a psyche disordered by manic excitation. This confrontation, taking place in the context of an awareness of his approaching death, promotes a moral and spiritual transformation which allows him, finally, to publicly confess his hitherto secret sin and embrace repentance before he dies.

The young daguerreotypist, Holgrave, has taken up residence in the House of the Seven Gables as a secret Maule nemesis whose purpose is to oversee Pyncheon destruction. His unexpected vigil with Jaffrey Pyncheon's corpse catalyzes an eruption of the unconscious in which he must come to terms with the baleful consequences of the long and tormented history of hostility between the Maules and Pyncheons and his role as an active participant in its finale. The transformation wrought by this encounter opens his heart to a loving bond with a Phoebe, a Pyncheon woman, and transmutes the severity of his social alienation and youthful radicalism.

In *The Blithedale Romance*, Zenobia keeps secret her dark past as she seeks a new life in the Blithedale community. However, her past overtakes her in the persons of her father, Old Moodie, half-sister, Priscilla and her former lover, Westervelt. In a confrontation with the buried traumas of her past after Old Moodie strips her of her fortune and Hollingsworth rejects her, Zenobia's unconscious identification with her dead mother prompts her to find release in suicide. In a variation of the pattern I am elucidating, it is Coverdale who is transformed by Zenobia's tragic death; his memoir, which constitutes the fabric of *The Blithedale Romance*, is in an act of mourning for the woman he loved and lost.

Not unlike Zenobia, in *The Marble Faun*, Miriam's secret past, in the form of the Model, overtakes her attempt at a *vita nuova* as an artist in Rome. At the edge of the Tarpeian Rock, while she is in a semi-conscious state, repressed destructive wishes toward the Model, her childhood sexual abuser, surface as his life is held in abeyance. Her reckoning with his death, as well as hers and Donatello's part in it, ushers in a far-reaching psychological transformation which is the substance of the remainder of the romance.

Finally, Hester's traumatic encounter with Dimmesdale's death on the scaffold enables a reconsideration of all that was involved in her life as a woman with the scarlet letter and its fateful consequences; the resulting psychological and spiritual transformation finds expression in her eventual return to Boston and resumption of the scarlet letter.

Even to those familiar with these works and the critical literature about them, these synopses sound unfamiliar and, perhaps, eccentric. The conclusions are not to be found in the vast critical literature that Hawthorne's four romances have inspired. As a matter of fact, they consistently contradict the consensus of contemporary critical judgments regarding these characters' fates. Why, the reader may reasonably ask, has this pattern of a crisis of the unconscious followed by momentous transformation not been apparent to the romances' readers, especially to those in the field of literary criticism? Hawthorne keeps the answer to that question hidden in an inside pocket: all of the confrontations with the unconscious and the transformations that result from them transpire within narrative gaps and are thus shuttered from the reader's view.

When the receptacles of his characters' haunted minds are flung open, Hawthorne shuts close the window upon them. The three days between Dimmesdale's return to his study, after his portentous reunion with Hester until his appearance in the Election Day procession, go unnarrated and the enormity of the internal changes that are at play are alluded to but not specified by the narrator: "That self was gone! Another man had returned out of the forest; a wiser one, with a knowledge of hidden mysteries which the simplicity of the former never could have reached" (p. 223). Precisely what are the hidden mysteries and what the wisdom and knowledge that will bring the minister to confession on the scaffold? The answers, never explicit in the text, lodge in the narrative gap.

Holgrave exclaims, "Could you but know, Phoebe, how it was with me, the hour before you came…A dark, cold, miserable hour! The presence of yonder dead man threw a great black shadow over everything; he made the universe, so far as my perception could reach, a scene of guilt, and of retribution more dreadful than guilt" (Hawthorne, 1962, Vol. 2, p. 306). How Holgrave traverses the wide psychological span from his reaction to seeing Jaffrey Pynchoen's dead body, who was, after all, a figure he despised, to, an hour later, a pervasive depression is not recorded. Moreover, it is left to the imagination why his dark vision is transmuted when, with Phoebe's appearance at the threshold, "The black moment became at once a blissful one" and the narrative gap finally ends with the spoken word, a declaration of love: "It must not pass without the spoken word. I love you!" (p. 306). Over the course of the hour vigil, Holgrave loses his aloofness and self-sufficiency in a near mental breakdown but emerges from the crisis as a more humane, vulnerable lover.

The thoughts that went through Zenobia's mind from the time she leaves Coverdale after their final colloquy until her act of suicide a short time later are shrouded in narrative silence. As a matter of fact, so much so that several critics have come to the wildly unsupportable conclusion that she did not kill herself but, instead, was murdered. These critics seem to agree with Silas Foster, who when confronted with her suicide, exclaims "What on earth should the young woman do that for?...There is some mistake about this, I tell you!" (Hawthorne, 1962, Vol. 3, pp. 230–231). Narrative gaps create interpretive dilemmas.

At the edge of the precipice, Miriam enters an altered state of consciousness in which: "her whole recollection of that wild moment, she beheld herself as in a dim show, and could not well distinguish what was done and suffered; so, not even whether she was really an actor and sufferer in the scene" (Hawthorne, 1962, Vol. 4, p. 171). Without the controls that inhere in consciousness, Miriam falls prey to the power of the unconscious, an experience which cannot be put into words. Donatello and Hilda will eventually fill in for her the narrative gap and its irrevocable result.

Finally, the narrator of *The Scarlet Letter*, who, as we have seen, lavishes attention on virtually every aspect of Hester's complex psychology, withdraws completely from her at the moment of Dimmesdale's death and does not bring her back to narrative life until some two decades later when she returns to Boston. What is Hester's reaction to her lover's death which thwarts the urgently anticipated escape from Puritan Boston and the end to seven years of suffering as an outcast? Of this there is no word in the text, only the disembodied statement, "in no long time after the physician's death, the wearer of the scarlet letter disappeared, and little Pearl with her" (p. 261). Hester's reaction to Dimmesdale's death needs to be read in the action she takes many years later. Sacvan Bercovitch (1988) underscores that Hester's decision occurs "at a certain missing point in the narrative, through an unrecorded process of introspection" (p. 631).

All the narrative gaps I will elucidate are of a particular species: in each instance, after a confrontation with the unconscious, the protagonist emerges from the gap and does something unexpected or seemingly out of character. Contrary to what we would anticipate, Dimmesdale, hitherto consumed by fear of exposure, publicly confesses; Hester returns to hated Boston; a self-possessed Holgrave implodes; the commanding Zenobia commits suicide; and Miriam falls in love with the man whose seemingly childlike affection she had earlier dismissed. In this way, Hawthorne evinces the double intentionality of leaving a gap and drawing attention to it. The gap creates a discontinuity in the psychological fabric of the narrative. The reader, unsettled by the sense of having missed something significant, must attempt to reweave the narrative "tear" through imagination and empathy. Thus, the reader becomes a participant-narrator of the transformation. In *The Marble Faun*, Hawthorne is specific as to the artist's need to recruit the reader: "A picture, however admirable the painter's art, and wonderful his power, requires of the spectator a surrender of himself, in due proportion with the miracle which has been wrought...There is always the necessity of helping out the painter's art with your own resources of sensibility and imagination" (p. 335).[2]

It would take more of a scholar than I could pretend to be to contextualize within literary history Hawthorne's use of this complex narrative strategy. It creates the double indemnity involving an eruption from the shadowy region of unconscious that is, as the same time, cloaked in a narrative gap. From his well-worn office chair, a psychoanalyst notices that through this narrative sleight of hand, Hawthorne assures that what is most consequential in the lives of his protagonists will be rendered obscure to the reader. What Hawthorne values, above all, for himself as an author, as expressed in the Custom-House introduction to *The Scarlet Letter*, he ensures for his characters: to "still keep the inmost Me behind its veil" (p. 4). When the repressed contents of protagonists' haunted minds are set free, Hawthorne veils them; at this time of their utmost vulnerability, there will be no voyeuristic violation of the sanctity of the human heart, the gravest sin in Hawthorne's moral hierarchy.

However protective it may be, the interpretive dilemma posed by this species of gaps, coming at crucial points in the narrative, is substantial. Sylvie Mathé (1992), in an extraordinarily thoughtful linguistic analysis of *The Scarlet Letter*, comments that "such a gap in the narrative process is a blurring of reality in which speculation comes to replace information and that withholding of information...partakes in the more general process of mystification by omission that characterizes Hawthorne's strategy. Gaps play a fundamental role in the deceptive tactics at work in the novel; crucial hermeneutic clues which would serve as central evidence in solving of the enigma, are thus withheld, making the task of interpreting, i.e. filling the gaps, a baffling aleatory one" (p. 626).

Hawthorne may baffle the reader, but the enigma, nonetheless, can be solved. We remember that Hawthorne holds out the necessity of his readers helping out his art with their resources of sensibility and imagination. I will attempt to show that the psychoanalytic method can help bridge the gaps so that a coherent narrative, which accounts for the relationship of the unconscious to the protagonist's transformation, can be credibly established. We must trust the tale and not the canny teller: things of great significance happen to these characters in these gaps and their fine-structure can be adduced and their meaning explored. The narration about them may stop but the characters' psyches do not. Referring to *The Scarlet Letter*, Bercovich (1988) is correct that "the silence surrounding Hester's conversion to the scarlet letter is deliberate on Hawthorne's part by forcing us to represent it for ourselves, by ourselves" (p. 631). In these chapters I attempt to represent the protagonists' conversions psychoanalytically.

The Psychoanalytic Narrative of a Fictional Character

Nancy Chodorow (1999) contrasts psychoanalytic epistemology and that of other humanistic disciplines. She writes: "Because psychological meaning is constitutive of internal and external perceptions and experiences from childhood on, the past is always drawn into the present" (p. 60) Chodorow considers psychoanalysis "first and foremost an account and theory of personal meaning" (p. 129), and its method is to unravel "the particularistic uniqueness of each individual psyche and life history" (p. 2). In its systematic consideration of "the power of feelings," which is the pithy title that Chodorow has given to her thought-provoking book, psychoanalysis distinguishes itself from other interpretive frameworks such as linguistic, historicist, and feminist, to name a few.

This volume is essentially a cross-discipline study which applies the insights of psychoanalysis to literary texts and therefore does not read like a work written within the genre of literary criticism. Like literary analysts, I pay scrupulous attention to the line by line reality of the text but unlike them, I am not primarily concerned with style, lexicon, syntax, structure, imagery pattern, rhetorical restraint, nor, on a larger scale, biography, the work's history, or its place within the spectrum of narrative styles. Michael Dunne (2004) would be correct to call this work an instance of "monological reading" which "involves tearing the web apart by sorting through the text" for passages which sustain the interpretive vantage (p. 25). My analytic method commits me to what a reader of an earlier draft called, and not kindly, "a surgical extraction" of the protagonists' psychological trajectory "from the fabric or design of the whole." Guilty as charged.

Following Chodorow's lead, in each chapter, I have constructed the protagonist's life narrative in its "particularistic uniqueness" in relation to determinative power of feelings. In these efforts, I am following a familiar technique of psychoanalytic treatment which employs a narrative method toward weaving the patient's association, memories, and dreams into a coherent pattern which includes conscious and unconscious elements. As Donald Spence (1982) contends, this pattern "allows us to make important discoveries about the patient's life and to make sense out of previously random events" (p. 21). Moreover, Spence emphasizes that Freud "made us aware of the persuasive power of a coherent narrative - in particular of the way in which an aptly chosen reconstruction can fill the gap between two apparently unrelated events and, in the process, make sense out of non-sense. There seems no doubt but that a well-constructed story possesses a narrative truth that is real and immediate and carries an important significance for the process of therapeutic change" (p. 21).

Indeed, in the treatment of neurotic illness, Freud was to find that when an analysand's forbidden wishes were most urgent, they were most forcefully repressed. A gap in the patient's associations signals a conflict over emerging unconscious desire. Thus efforts of the analysand's psyche to suppress the emergence of the "buried prisoners and ghosts" of the haunted mind is a very familiar scenario for the clinical psychoanalyst; in fact, it is the *modus operandi* by which he earns a living, hour after hour. It is not surprising, then, that a psychoanalyst would be particularly alert to Hawthorne's strategy of narrative gaps at times of greatest unconscious force and seek to employ the psychoanalytic method in order to analyze them. And perhaps, you will eventually allow, a psychoanalyst may be uniquely poised to unravel their mysteries.

Hawthorne, who strews the path to understanding his characters with many obstacles, the narrative gap being one, also serves as a guide in this pursuit by setting out the roadmap, as it were, to reach the goal. In relation to Chillingworth's attempt to "know" Dimmesdale, and discover the secret underlying his illness, the narrator of *The Scarlet Letter* offers the following extraordinarily salient wisdom:

> A man burdened with a secret should especially avoid the intimacy of his physician. If the latter possesses native sagacity, and a nameless something more, –let us call it intuition; if he show no intrusive egotism, nor disagreeably prominent characteristics of his own; if he have the power, which must be born with him, to bring his mind into such affinity with his patient's, that this last shall unawares have spoken what he imagines himself only to have thought; if such revelations be received without tumult, and acknowledged not so often by an uttered sympathy, as by silence, an inarticulate breath, and here and there a word, to indicate that all is understood; if, to these qualifications of a confidant be joined the advantages afforded by his recognized character as a physician; –then, at some inevitable moment, will the soul of the sufferer be dissolved, and flow forth in a dark, but transparent stream, bringing all its mysteries into the daylight (p. 124).

For Hawthorne, empathy informed by intuition and sagacity, and undistorted by an intrusive personal agenda, constitutes the capacity for an understanding of another being. In this Hawthorne presages what Freud and generations of psychoanalysts who followed him arrived at about the ideal therapeutic relationship between analyst and analysand. In one sweep of the pen, as it were, Hawthorne establishes the theoretical ground for the position of psychoanalytic neutrality, empathic listening, evenly hovering attention, and attunement to countertransference as crucial parameters in the analytic situation.

Hawthorne, I believe, would have us bring our minds and hearts into close affinity with his protagonists during their periods of intense vulnerability, thus to participate in their profound transformations. Empathy, intuition and sagacity, Hawthorne tells us, will provide the reader with "crucial hermeneutical clues" which serve as central evidence in solving the enigma posed by a narrative gap; for these efforts the reader will be privileged to apprehend the mysteries of the protagonist's soul as it is brought "into the daylight."[3]

That said, a psychoanalytic investigation of a fictional character is a perilous matter. Psychoanalytic technique was devised for and generated by the clinical situation, a living dynamic between analyst and analysand. In this context, the analyst's interpretation of the unconscious can be revised and modified in light of the analysand's emotional reactions and memories generated by the interpretation. In dialectical fashion, involving the unconscious of both analysand and analyst, mutual construction of the analysand's psychic reality has its best chance of arriving at psychological truth. The analyst inevitably will intrude his own unconscious contents onto the analysand's associations. Only by constant attunement to his own feeling states and the analysand's reactions to interpretations, can this intrusion, technically termed counter-transference, be taken into account and its influence on the construction and understanding of the analysand's psychic reality be diminished.

Such precautions are scarcely possible in the analysis of a fictional character. The character can neither confirm nor repel our interpretation, nor can the deceased author. Memories of childhood, which is a central focus of psychoanalytic treatment, cannot, of course, be evoked. When, in *The Marble Faun,* the Model says to Miriam, the "later thraldom in which I hold you… [has] scarcely made your cheek paler than I saw in your childhood, Miriam" (p. 94), Hawthorne has invited the reader to imagine Miriam's childhood and the Model's part in it; the character can take it no further. My imaginings about Miriam's relationship to the Model, discussed in Chapter 4, prompted one literary critic to censoriously comment: "The author forgets much of the time that Miriam and the others are artistic creations, products of Hawthorne's imagination, not actual human beings with actual childhoods." Call it an occupational hazard, if you will. Alas, the unconscious mind of the reader is always engaged by a literary work and will, of necessity, color understanding, and interpretation. Our subjectivity is always in tension with attempts at objectivity.

In his searching essay, "Mind in the Modern World," Lionel Trilling (1981) expresses this dilemma in relation to the efforts of literary criticism toward objectivity. Drawing on Matthew Arnold's characterization of literature as a "criticism of life" and the definition of literary criticism as the effort to "see the object as in itself it really is," Trilling views objectivity as "the respect we give to the object as object, as it exists apart from us" (p. 122). Furthermore, the "ideal of objectivity requires only that, before the personal response is given, the effort to see the object as in itself it really is be well and truly made" (p. 122). This ideal is virtually identical with that which informs the psychoanalytic situation.

While an analysand is not a fictional character and Hawthorne's characters are not analysands, a bridge between the wide difference in their species is created by the "truth of the human heart" which is encoded in their respective psyches. Indeed, this type of effort is possible only because Hawthorne provides so much in-depth psychological data about the character. These data can be organized and sequenced into a coherent psychological narrative of substantial explanatory power. As in the clinical situation, my analysis proceeds inductively, from observation to inference and finally, to interpretation. Paul Keegan (2017) is accurate in his judgment that "[p]sychoanalysis sets out to show rather than tell, and to redress the immemorial injury of speaking for the subject" (p. 5). My reliance on extensive quotations from the text is in the service of rendering a more objective portrait by letting Hawthorne's protagonists, as much as possible, speak for themselves. In this approach, I ask of the reader something akin to the narrator's appeal in *The House of the Seven Gables*: "The author needs great faith in his reader's sympathy; else he must hesitate to give details so minute, and incidents apparently so trifling, as are essential to make up the idea of this garden-life" (p. 150).

A disclaimer is in order: in these chapters I select, order, and interpret data congenial to the epistemological assumptions of Freud's psychoanalysis. Other psychoanalytic perspectives, and there are many, would involve other emphases which would undoubtedly yield a different order of interpretations. However, what I say about a psychoanalytic perspective is equally true of the text viewed from other organizing perspectives be they historical, linguistic, philosophical, allegorical, theological, or feminist, to name just a few. Every discipline is intrinsically limited by the universe of its epistemological assumptions. Joel Pfister (1991) is concerned that "[p]sychoanalysis tends to foreclose our consideration of social and historical processes" (p. 86). The analyses that follows aim not to foreclose other perspectives but, by giving expression to a distinctive psychoanalytic voice, to complement them and to invite response in the ongoing critical conversation about Hawthorne's protagonists.

It is my conviction that the greatness and perdurance of Hawthorne's romances lie in the inexhaustible ways that truths emanate from them in every aspect, like multitudinous beams of light from a central source. To extend the metaphor, every critical approach to the text captures but one beam in a prism and is refracted according to the prism's interpretive index. Taking into account the variety of disciplines and the evolving historical circumstances and cultural assumptions in which they are rooted, not to mention the influence of individual characteristics of the interpreter, the number of prisms and thus the interpretations they yield are virtually unlimited. Any interpreter of Hawthorne's romances who claims to have discovered something new about the text is humbled in the face of these considerations.

Which Hawthorne

A Psychoanalyst in the Hawthorne Literary Criticism Wars

Although I draw on the works of other critics about whose work there are instances of both accord and disagreement that are detailed in the individual chapters, the psychoanalytic interpretations of the characters in this volume are largely *sui generis*. I have kept my eyes open to the texts, followed my instincts as a psychoanalyst and have reported what I saw. So far as I can tell, I have allowed empathy to be informed by intuition and by whatever sagacity I possess after years as a clinician; I am not aware of a personal agenda which has distorted my visual field. I have attempted to strive toward Trilling's ideal to "see the object as in itself it really is": an understanding of Hawthorne's characters as he inscribed them in the text has been the sole desideratum of this cross-discipline study.

It came as a surprise, and not a welcome one, to discover that my efforts regarding the romances were very much out of step with contemporary trends in Hawthorne criticism. A relative, who is a professor of literature, candidly warned me, "Close reading and psychoanalysis are not in favor." Indeed, in my survey of the critical literature of last few decades, there was scant attention paid to the psychology that Hawthorne so carefully invested in his characters. It seemed that there was a general consensus that the characters' psychology, if germane at all, had already been thoroughly investigated, documented, and substantiated. There was seemingly nothing left to say about the matter. Frederick Crews's *The Sins of the Father: Hawthorne's Psychological Themes* (1996) was considered both "ground-breaking" and definitive. Unfortunately, it is a deeply flawed work. Not without flashes of insight, Crews, overall, has not the patience to attend systematically to Hawthorne's text but, in my opinion, imposes on it interpretations that are idiosyncratic and unduly influenced by the author's prejudices and animosities, attributes that are inimical to the psychoanalytic spirit and method. In a caricature of early applications of Freudian theory to literary interpretation, Crews is out to prove that an unresolved Oedipus complex lies behind all Hawthorne's work and that the author was afflicted with ever-mounting anxiety over incest which eventually overtook his efforts to write fiction. Crews eventually retracted the entirety of this book. Nevertheless, Crews's work was widely read and quoted, but neither built upon nor challenged as it was published at the beginning of an era of growing, decades-long critical disaffection with Freud. Psychological analyses of Hawthorne's romances virtually disappeared from the scholarly literature. The retreat from psychological investigation of Hawthorne's work was premature as it left unsolved mysteries which lie at the core of each of his four romances.

David Greven considers *The Fragility of Manhood: Hawthorne, Freud, and the Politics of Gender* (2014) to be "the first avowedly psychoanalytic study [of Hawthorne] since Crews's" (p. 71). In it, Greven recasts Freudian and Lacanian literary theory to interpret Hawthorne's depiction of masculinity. He advances as the chief claim of the book that "Nathaniel Hawthorne's work consistently evokes the core themes of the Narcissus myth" (p. 24); in doing so, Greven consciously upends the primacy of place in Hawthorne's psychology that Crews had ascribed, instead, to the Oedipus myth. By engaging various psychoanalytic theories of narcissism, Greven pursues, with rhetorical agility, the themes of Narcissus to help explain "the startling discrepancy between the nineteenth-century model of hegemonic or code masculinity and Hawthorne's representation of it," a discrepancy which he believes is the source of "Hawthorne's anguish" (p. 18). In arriving at his conclusions, Greven draws on elements of Hawthorne's fiction and non-fiction, biography, and cultural history. Despite a common interest in Freudian theory, Greven's volume and mine have virtually no points of overlap in purpose or content.

He utilizes a wide-angle lens to encompass broad intellectual terrain; my lens is telescopic and, in the tradition of the psychoanalytic method, is constrained by a persistent focus on the narrative sequence that Hawthorne provides and what it tells about the inner lives of each of five of his protagonists. The differences in our books can be encompassed by the single observation that *The Fragility of Manhood* makes scarce mention of Dimmesdale, Hester, Holgrave, Zenobia, or Miriam, nor does it allude to their psychological crises and transformations which form the warp and woof of my study. Psychoanalysis's tent is commodious: psychoanalytic studies of the same author may be situated so far apart in it that they do not have occasion to interact with one other.[4]

If the settled critical wisdom about the protagonists happened to be accurate, so much the better; I had no wish to devote the next several years to writing interpretations that were available in the literature. This was not to be the case, as there was a significant disparity between the results of my analyses of the characters' fates and those that appeared in the academic literature. As a matter of fact, I had strong disagreements with many prevailing judgments and experienced cognitive dissonance when I encountered them in the literature. I mention here some salient examples which I will elaborate upon in the chapters: a consensus of critics contend that Hester does not return to Boston and resume the scarlet letter "of her own free will" (p. 263); instead, it is Hawthorne who, against the impulses of her authentic self, "brings his heroine back...out of a desire to punish her" (Tassi, 1998, p. 34) and thus "does violence to the living character whom he had created" (Carpenter, 1988, p. 68). In the end, so critics conclude, Dimmesdale does not experience that his former "self was gone!" but remains "an unreconstructed narcissist intent of the last dose of celebrity" (Millington, 1992, p. 85) and, regarding his Election Sermon, even though there was "united testimony, never had a man spoken in so wise, so high and so holy a spirit," (Hawthorne, Vol. 1, 1962, p. 248) one critic can nevertheless assert that the minister is a man whose "impotencies—sexual, emotional, moral and verbal—infiltrate every area of his life" (Valenti, 2014, p. 24). As a consequence of his encounter with Death, it is not most significant that Holgrave has found in Phoebe the "only possibility of happiness" (Vol. 2, p. 306), but, critics concur, that he has "lost himself in the darkened parlor" and will "abandon his art" (Baym, 1970, pp. 593–594). Zenobia is not a "radiant presence" who embodies Nature's "fairest handiwork" (Vol. 3, p. 245) but, quite the opposite, is likened to a "Medusan harlot" (Greven, 2012, p. 125). Although Kenyon describes Miriam as possessing "rich gifts of heart and mind, a suggestive power, a magnetic influence, a sympathetic knowledge" (Vol. 4, p. 321), she is judged "an overblown, oversexed, aggressive woman" (Crews, 1996, p. 215). There is a great deal at stake here: whatever a critic's interpretive bent, a disregard for psychology may lead to serious misreading and faulty interpretations in these densely psychologically-wrought works and thus do a disservice to Hawthorne's literary purpose. It is true: Hawthorne's signature ambiguities, ambivalences, and ironies, as well as the narrative gaps discussed in this volume, are challenging; however, it would seem that these difficulties do not justify discarding the text in favor of wild surmise, but are a call for granting close psychological reading with substantial hermeneutic authority. Hawthorne would have us lean in, not away.

The resemblance in kind of these radically counter-textual readings raises a different question: is there also a prevailing critical agenda which is strongly coloring these critics' interpretive efforts? Stated in Hawthorne's terms, do the recent critics of his romances possess "intrusive egotism or disagreeably prominent characteristics" which prevent them from establishing an affinity with his protagonists? In pursuing an answer to this vexing question, I had unwittingly entered the labyrinth of the Hawthorne literary criticism wars.

In that journey I was to find my bearings in Lionel Trilling's notable essay, "Our Hawthorne" (1964). Trilling calls attention to the way cultural assumptions have had a shaping influence on critical views of Hawthorne. He points out that Henry James' Hawthorne is distinctly different from the tragic Hawthorne of his own era whose "quick response to the non-rational, his lively awareness of the primitive and chthonic, of the dark roots of life, does not deflect the naturalistic and humanistic tendency of his mind" (p. 456).

Gordon Hutner's article, "Whose Hawthorne" (2004), is a critique, and not a generous one, of Trilling's essay in which he presents a chilling update to some of its conclusions. Hutner finds that in the intervening fifty years there has been what amounts to a seismic change in American critical judgments of Hawthorne in that:"[his] appeal to the idea of the interiority and the complexity of human motives, his worries about the risks of individualism and the cost of freedom, his skepticism about worldly success, the obduracy of the material world, all seem [...] much too irrelevant" (p. 258). The Hawthorne of today, "our" Hawthorne, "who sometimes no longer matters at all" is, in Hutner's further assessment of prevailing critical judgments including his own, "an author whose great purpose is to expose his own inauthenticity and debility, thereby unveiling the corruption of the critical world that enshrined him" (p. 259). What is relevant to Hutner and his cohorts, however, is that Hawthorne "too little prepares us for the great inequities of the mid-century: slavery and rights of women, the rights of labor; instead, his example upholds the structures whereby those moral wrongs are promoted...At the worse, this Hawthorne is a writer too often racist and sexist, a writer who trusted too little in the very powers of sympathy he exalted and who may well owe his stature to a network of publishing friends and influential critics" (p. 262).

As if being racist, sexist, and an unsympathetic perpetrator of a system of injustice by which he undeservedly achieved literary fame were not quite enough with which to tarnish Hawthorne, Hutner engages in summarizing fantastical *ad hominem* denigrations: "Hawthorne was a damaged young man, perhaps sexually abused, who yearned for bourgeois respectability that his marriage to Sophia Peabody was supposed to certify. In the past he was understood as Byronic; today, Hawthorne is more likely to be read for the ways his vision embraces masochism, fear of women, and homosexual panic" (p. 263). As the host of such overwhelming "inauthenticity and debility," one wonders how Hawthorne could have held his head up long enough to write *The Scarlet Letter.* True to the manifesto he outlines, Hutner uses a degraded Hawthorne for the purpose of "unveiling the corruption" of Trilling's critical world because it had "enshrined him." It was, after all, Trilling and New Criticism who, Hutner contends, assimilated Hawthorne's tragic sense for the purpose of "accommodating a generation's need to obscure complicity with guilt and corruption, its unacknowledged association with bourgeois conformity or material well-being" (p. 253).

It is not my purpose to deconstruct this jumbled screed which lacks even a pretense of scholarly restraint. Larry J. Reynold's rigorous historical study, *Devils & Rebels: The Making of Hawthorne's Damned Politics* (2010), challenges misconceptions about the cast of Hawthorne's political thought which, he concludes, was founded in Christian pacifism not moral turpitude.[5] George Hutchinson's recent *Facing the Abyss: American Literature and Culture in the 1940s* (2018) offers a thoughtful discussion of the historical context and contributions of Trilling and New Criticism. It is important to acknowledge, however, that Hutner is an accomplished Hawthorne scholar, whose *Secrets and Sympathy: Forms of Disclosure in Hawthorne's Novels,* published in 1988, is the product of serious and systematic consideration of the psychological universe inscribed by Hawthorne in his romances. A consideration of "the complexity of human motives," a foundational assumption of his book, has somehow become irrelevant for him by 2004. Moreover, in this work Hutner does not utter a word of concern for the social agenda that he insists Hawthorne should have addressed in his fiction over one-hundred twenty-five years earlier. There is more than a whiff of intellectual hypocrisy in Hutner's diatribe; apparently sometime after 1988 he quaffed a particularly potent formula of Kool-Aid which both incited self-righteousness and dulled self-reflection.

We will find our out way of this dark corridor of the labyrinth presently. In Hutner's heated rhetoric it is not hard to locate prevailing critical biases, the *fons et origo* of an "intrusive egotism and disagreeably prominent characteristics," which compromise these critics' capacity for emotional affinity with Hawthorne's protagonists so that they are not present when, "*at some inevitable moment, will the soul of the sufferer be dissolved, and flow forth in a dark, but transparent stream, bringing all its mysteries into the daylight*" (Vol. 1, p. 124, emphasis added).

As it relates to interpreting the romances, Hutner alludes to two of the narrative gaps I will be analyzing: "Hawthorne came to signify to contemporary readers the limits of American democracy, the willingness to make peace with the forces of corruption, *as in Hester's return or Holgrave's end,* this new recognition has led to Hawthorne's undoing, maybe even his passing" (Hutner, 2004, p. 258, emphasis added). This "new recognition" is, in fact, a blindness which results from relying on interpretations that have been made in the service of ideology, and thus, constitute a failure "to see the object as in itself it really is." "Hester's return" and "Holgrave's end," my analyses demonstrate, in no way "make peace with the forces of corruption" in American democracy; quite the opposite, they are statements of strong moral purpose by two of the finest fictional characters about whom American democracy can boast. Such crucial interpretive inaccuracies, piled upon one other, which bend literary meaning to the service of a social agenda, however admirable the agenda, will eventually be the "undoing" and "passing" of this wave of Hawthorne criticism. The report of Hawthorne's literary death was an exaggeration.

Roy Harvey Pearce, an editor of the twenty-three-volume *Centenary Edition of the Works of Nathaniel Hawthorne*, gets it just right. In the Introductory Note to a book of centenary essays (1964), in which Trilling's "Our Hawthorne" is the culmination, he states on behalf of all the editors, "However rooted in historical understanding, critical studies, we decided, would not in their very nature have the staying power of the texts we should establish." Hawthorne's critics, as Trilling underscored in "Our Hawthorne," come and go, bringing with them and then passing out of existence, their particular societal struggles, anxieties, needs, and biases. *The Scarlet Letter, The House of the Seven Gables, The Blithedale Romance,* and *The Marble Faun* are not for an age, but for all time. The narrator of *The House of the Seven Gables* says it best: "But we strive in vain to put it into words. No adequate expression of the beauty and profound pathos with which it impresses us, is attainable" (Vol. 2, p. 142).

Although it is not a central purpose, this work also seeks to redress, in its way, the damage done to Hawthorne's literary reputation over the past several decades. There is a great deal at stake for the American literary tradition and its students as such a diminished estimation of Hawthorne's oeuvre constitutes a substantial cultural loss. Through close psychological reading, this study attempts to bring the reader back to the texts that Hawthorne wrote and draw attention to the urgent moral and spiritual conflicts that envelop the protagonists, conflicts that underpin all movement toward human liberation.

Hawthorne's exquisitely subtle and complex renderings of these conflicts engaged my psychoanalytic imagination and allowed me to sustain a solitary effort in an unaccustomed scholarly discipline whose rigors were very different from those of the clinical situation. Through it all Hawthorne was an inspiring companion who, in abundant fulfillment of Joseph Conrad's vision of the artist's mission, spoke to me, as he has to generations of readers, of "the subtle but invincible conviction of solidarity that knits together the loneliness of innumerable hearts, to the solidarity in dreams, in joy, in sorrow, in aspirations, in illusions, in hope, in fear, which binds men to each other, which binds together all humanity—the dead to the living and the living to the unborn" (Conrad, 1921, pp. viii–ix).

Notes

1. A statement about Hawthorne's imagining of death frames the first chapter of Roberta Weldon's interesting volume, *Hawthorne, Gender and Death: Christianity and Its Discontents* (2008): "In a notebook entry of 1836, Nathaniel Hawthorne imagines death not in the more conventional images of the grim reaper or the devil but as 'a great parent' that 'comes and sweeps them all through one darksome portal, –all his children' (8:22–23)" (p. 13).
2. As a tribute to its importance, Hawthorne makes the same point on two other occasions. When the aesthetic company peruses a portfolio of drawings by the Old Masters, the narrator comments on the "divinity of the first sketch" when compared to the finished picture: "The charm lay partly in their very imperfections; for this is suggestive, and sets the imagination at work" (Vol. 4, p. 138). Hilda later elaborates on this same theme: "'there is a class of spectator whose sympathy will help them to see the Perfect through a mist of imperfection. Nobody, I think, ought to read poetry, or look at pictures or statues, who cannot find a great deal more in them than the poet or artist has actually expressed. Their highest merit is their suggestiveness'" (Hawthorne, 1962, p. 379).
3. As the reader will discover, my analyses of the protagonists draw almost exclusively on the abundant "crucial hermeneutical clues" offered by the romances' texts and do not build on formulations of Hawthorne's personal psychology. Gloria C. Ehrlich's *Family Themes and Hawthorne's Fiction: The Tenacious Web* (1984) pays scrupulous attention to Hawthorne's early psychological development and attempts to correlate his psychology with the psychological themes of his fiction. However, her admirable book does not provide insights into the particular crises and transformations that are my subject. Stepping back from the specifics of Ehrlich's contribution and other studies of that ilk, I would like to say that for this psychoanalyst it is axiomatic that the writer's past will profoundly influence in manifold ways what eventually appears on the written page. However, the sorting, selecting, sequencing, interpreting, and representing, for aesthetic and literary purpose, what is, after all, an infinitesimal fraction of past experience occurs through unimaginably complex processes that are far beyond the ken of psychoanalytic theory. Freudian psychoanalysis falters at the gates of artistic creativity. *The Scarlet Letter* is brimming with vitality, power and mystery compared to which Hawthorne psycho-biographies, however informative, are tedious and uninspired. Since I believe it, I will say it: all that the reader needs know about Hawthorne's psyche inheres in the pages of his romances. TS Eliot put it this way; "I do not say that poetry is not 'autobiographical': but this autobiography is written by a foreign man in a foreign tongue and can never be translated." Quoted from "Emily of Fire & Violence" (Paul Keegan, 2020, p. 18). The question posed by Yeats' famous couplet expresses my sentiment: *O body swayed to music, O brightening glance,/How can we know the dancer from the dance?*
4. Greven's interpretation of Hester's return to Boston is found in the last chapter of his *Gender Protest and Same-Sex Desire in Antebellum American Literature* (2014) and will be considered in Chapter 6 of this volume.
5. David S. Reynolds did not seem to incorporate the insights offered in *Devils and Rebels* into his Keynote Talk, "Hawthorne and Democratic Politics" delivered at the Nathaniel Hawthorne Society Conference (Stowe, Vermont, June 3, 2016). His address, which went no further than a reiteration of a familiar set of grievances against what has been cast as Hawthorne's politics, struck, to this listener, a decidedly sour note.

References

Baym, N. (1970). The Failure of the Artist-Hero. *The Journal of English and German Philology, 69.*

Bercovitch, S. (1988). The A-Politics of Ambiguity in *The Scarlet Letter. New Literary History, 19*(3), 631.

Bloom, H. (2004). *Bloom's Major Literary Characters: Hester Prynne.* In H. Bloom (Ed.), New York: Chelsea House.

Carpenter, F. (1988). Scarlet A Minus. In D. B. Kesterson, & G. K. Hall (Eds.), *Critical Essays on Hawthorne's The Scarlet Letter.*

Chodorow, N. J. (1999). *The Power of Feelings.* New Haven: Princeton.

Conrad, J. (1921). *The Nigger of the Narcissus: A Tale of the Forecastle.* New York and Toronto: Doubleday, Page & Co.

Crews, F. (1996). *The Sins of the Father: Hawthorne's Psychological Themes.* New York: Oxford University Press.

Dunne, M. (2004). Tearing the Web Apart: Resisting Monological Interpretations in *The Marble Faun. South Atlantic Review, 69.*

Ehrlich, G. C. (1984). *Family Themes and Hawthorne's Fiction: The Tenacious Web.* New Brunswick, NJ: Rutgers University Press.

Greven, D. (2012). *The Fragility of Manhood: Hawthorne, Freud and the Politics of Gender.* Columbus: Ohio State University Press.

Hawthorne, N. (1974). Endicott and the Red Cross. In W. Charvat (Ed.), *The Centenary Edition of the Works of Nathaniel Hawthorne* (Vol. 9). Columbus: Ohio University State Press.

Hawthorne, N. (1962a).*The Blithedale Romance.* In W. Charvat (Ed.), *The Centenary Edition of the Works of Nathaniel Hawthorne* (Vol. 3). Columbus: Ohio State University Press.

Hawthorne, N. (1962b). *The House of the Seven Gables.* In W. Charvat (Ed.), *The Centenary Edition of the Works of Nathaniel Hawthorne* (Vol. 2).Columbus: Ohio University State Press.

Hawthorne, N. (1962c). *The Marble Faun.* In W. Charvat (Ed.), *The Centenary Edition of the Works of Nathaniel Hawthorne* (Vol. 4). Columbus: Ohio State University Press.

Hawthorne, N. (1962d). *The Scarlet Letter.* In W. Charvat (Ed.), *The Centenary Edition of the Works of Nathaniel Hawthorne* (Vol. 1). Columbus: Ohio State University Press.

Hawthorne, N. (1974). The Haunted Mind. In W. Charvat (Ed.), *The Centenary Edition of the Works of Nathaniel Hawthorne* (Vol. 9). Columbus: Ohio University State Press.

Hutchinson, G. (2018). *Facing the Abyss: American Literature and Culture in the 1940s.* New York: Columbia University Press.

Hutner, G. (2004). Whose Hawthorne. In R. H. Millington (Ed.), *The Cambridge Companion to Nathaniel Hawthorne.* Cambridge: Cambridge University Press.

James, H. (1879). *Hawthorne.* London: MacMillan.

Keegan, P. (2017). From Shtetl to Boulevard. *The London Review of Books, 39.*

Keegan, P. (2020). Emily of Fire & Violence. *The London Review of Books, 42*(20).

Mathé, S. (1992). The Reader May Not Choose: Oxymoron as Central Figure on Hawthorne's Strategy of Immunity from Choice in The Scarlet Letter. *Style, 26*(4), 604–633.

Matthiessen, F. O. (1941). *American Renaissance: Art and Expression in the Age of Emerson and Whitman.* New York: Oxford University Press.
Milder, R. (2014). *The Scarlet Letter*–Again??? *Nathaniel Hawthorne Review, 40,* 105–122.
Millington, R. H. (1992). *Practicing Romance: Narrative Form and Cultural Engagement in Hawthorne's Fiction.* Princeton: Princeton University Press.
Pfister, J. (1991). *The Production of Personal Life: Class, Gender, and the Psychological in Hawthorne's Fiction.* Stanford, CA: Stanford University Press.
Reynolds, D. S. (2016). Keynote Talk: Hawthorne and Democratic Politics. Nathaniel Hawthorne Society Conference. Stowe, Vermont.
Reynolds, L. J. (2010). *Devils and Rebels: The Making of Hawthorne's Damned Politics.* Ann Arbor: University of Michigan Press.
Spence, D. (1982). *Narrrative Truth and Historical Truth: Meaning and Interpretation in Psychoanalysis.* New York: WW Norton.
Tassi, N. (1998). Prisons: Sex, Intellect, and Gender in *The Scarlet Letter. CEA Critic, 60*(3), 23–36.
Trilling, L. (1964). Our Hawthorne. In R. H. Pearce (Ed.), *Hawthorne Centenary Essays.* Columbus, Ohio: Ohio State University Press.
Trilling, L. (1981). Mind in the Modern World. In D. Trilling (Ed.), *The Last Decade: Essays and Reviews, 1965–1975.* New York and London: Harcourt, 100–128
Valenti, P. D. (2014). 'Then, All Was Spoken!' What 'The Custom-House' and The Scarlet Letter Disclose. *Nathaniel Hawthorne Review, 40.*
Weldon, R. (2008). *Hawthorne, Gender and Death: Christianity and Its Discontents.* New York: Palgrave MacMillan.

2 The Transformations of Arthur Dimmesdale in *The Scarlet Letter*: "That self was gone!"

After his fateful encounter with Hester in the forest and nightmarish walk through town, Arthur Dimmesdale finally reaches his study where he experiences relief and refuge amongst his familiar surroundings. At the same time, he becomes aware of a momentous internal change that has decisively transformed him since he left his dwelling two days earlier:

> Here he had studied and written; here, gone through fast and vigil, and had come forth half alive; here, striven to pray; here, borne a hundred thousand agonies! …He knew it was himself, the thin and white-cheeked minister, who had done and suffered these things, and written thus far into the Election Sermon! But he seemed to stand apart, and eye this former self with scornful, pitying, but half-envious curiosity. That self was gone! Another man had returned out of the forest; a wiser one; with a knowledge of hidden mysteries which the simplicity of the former never could have reached. A bitter kind of knowledge that! (Hawthorne, 1962, Vol. 1, pp. 222–223).

The reader's curiosity is aroused by these remarkable assertions: what is the knowledge, which hidden mysteries and what is the wisdom that Dimmesdale has acquired? What of himself, viewed as he is "standing apart" does he see? Who is this new man? The narrator, who has spared the reader no detail of Dimmesdale's mental deterioration, is silent as to the mental processes involved in this transformation. Although this change is not expressed in words, it is revealed in The Reverend's subsequent actions: the dismissal of Chillingworth as his physician, the delivery of an inspired and authentic Election Sermon, a confession of guilt on the scaffold, and the public acknowledgment of Pearl as his daughter. None of these actions, which are all contrary to the reader's expectations, is possible under the aegis of his former passive and paralyzed self. That self is now truly gone.

It is no secret that *The Scarlet Letter* is a psychological novel: word for word, chapter after chapter, scarcely a serious work of literature devotes itself more to the inner life, and its conflicts than Hawthorne's first romance. The small, claustrophobic Puritan colony, with its stark rules of conduct and abundant opportunity for voyeuristic zeal, provides a narrow, shallow, and brilliantly lit stage against which the inner lives of the intensely entangled, conflicted, and tormented characters play out. Their secrets, always under pressure of exposure, set them apart from their community, from each other, and from themselves. Under the burden of psychic strain, each character is prone to forms of psychological deterioration. Although it is true of all the protagonists, Arthur Dimmesdale best exemplifies the judgment expressed in *The House of the Seven Gables,* "For, what other dungeon is so dark as one's own heart! What jailer so inexorable as one's self!" (Hawthorne, 1962, Vol. 2, p. 169). Indeed, *The Scarlet Letter* details the exacting trials of a man who "...above all things else...loathed his miserable self!" (Vol. 1, p. 144) but who ultimately finds release in his final scene where he "stood with a flush of triumph in his face, as one who, in the crisis of acutest pain, had won a victory" (p. 255).

What is the psychology of this momentous transformation? It is a question that comes naturally to the mind of a psychoanalyst to whom psychological change is not only of interest but a desideratum of psychoanalytic treatment. Although an analysand is not a fictional character, and Dimmesdale is not an analysand, a bridge between the wide differences in their species is created by the "truth of the human heart," valorized in the Preface to *The House of the Seven Gables,* which is encoded in their respective psyches. A cross-disciplinary study which applies a psychoanalytic perspective to a literary work is only possible because Hawthorne provides an abundance of data for psychoanalytic inquiry, namely, the intricate interweaving of the character's conscious and unconscious motivations and their vicissitudes. These data can be organized and sequenced into a coherent psychological narrative of substantial explanatory power; the psychology of Dimmesdale's transformation will be interpreted in the light of this narrative. As in the clinical situation, my analysis proceeds inductively, from observation to inference and finally, to interpretation. Paul Keegan (2017) is accurate in his judgment that "Psychoanalysis sets out to show rather than tell, and to redress the immemorial injury of speaking for the subject" (p. 5). My reliance on extensive quotations from the text is in the service of rendering a more objective portrait by letting Dimmesdale, as much as possible, speak for himself. In this approach, I ask of the reader something akin to the narrator's appeal in *The House of the Seven Gables*: "The author needs great faith in his reader's sympathy; else he must hesitate to give details so minute, and incidents apparently so trifling, as are essential to make up the idea of this garden-life" (Vol. 2, p. 150).

In this chapter I select, order, and interpret data congenial to the epistemological assumptions of Freudian psychoanalysis. Other psychoanalytic perspectives, and there are many, would involve other emphases and undoubtedly would yield different orders of interpretations. This is also true of approaching Dimmesdale's transformation from other organizing perspectives be they historical, allegorical, linguistic, philosophical, theological, or feminist, to name just a few. Every discipline is intrinsically limited by the universe of its epistemological assumptions. It is my conviction that the greatness and perdurance of *The Scarlet Letter* lies in the inexhaustible ways that truths emanate from it, like multitudinous beams of light from a central source. To extend the metaphor, every critical approach to the text captures but one beam in a prism and is refracted according to the prism's interpretive index. It is not within the scope of this essay to situate the conclusions of my analysis with those of other interpretive modes, but to circumscribe the contribution as yet another voice in the ongoing critical conversation about Hawthorne's Dimmesdale.

A psychoanalytic framework in the tradition of Freud was largely prefigured by Hawthorne. The prototype for the system of psychology which informs *The Scarlet Letter* was put forth with succinctness and force in Hawthorne's early sketch "The Haunted Mind" (1835) which anticipates, with uncanny accuracy, Freud's topographic model of the mind in its delineation of the terrain of the id, ego, and superego and the forces which govern their interaction.[1] Magisterially, the narrator of "The Haunted Mind" generalizes about the very nature of the psyche:

> In the depth of every heart, is a tomb and a dungeon, though the lights, the music, and the revelry above, may cause us to forget their existence, and the buried ones or prisoners whom they hide. But sometimes, and oftenest at midnight, those dark recepticles are flung wide open (Hawthorne, 1974, Vol. IX, p. 306).

For both Hawthorne and Freud, the unconscious is a dynamic force which always presses upward toward expression; stored as unconscious, affect-laden memory, the past forever haunts the present. At certain crucial times, the hidden contents of the haunted mind may flood into consciousness and produce far-reaching disruption of psychic functioning. Such a confrontation with the repressed is precisely what Dimmesdale experiences in the aftermath of his encounter with Hester in the forest, and is a precondition for the transformation which follows from it.

My analysis of Dimmesdale finds that this transformation is the final of three that he undergoes in *The Scarlet Letter.* The first, which has not been adequately appreciated in the critical literature but is central to understanding his subsequent psychological course, begins some months before the opening scene of the romance. The Reverend Dimmesdale is a promising young man of outstanding intellectual and religious accomplishment whose particular psychic structure cannot bear the burden of guilt consequent to adultery. By the opening of the story, he has already fallen ill with a severe neurotic illness which reduces him from man of stature and dignity to a pathetic character whose deterioration into a state of morbid depression is detailed over the course of the novel. The second transformation, seven years later, is from melancholia to mania; it is an immediate result of his encounter with Hester in the forest, which temporarily frees him from the oppression of a relentlessly punitive superego. But the manic state is short lived; the third and most consequential transformation transpires after Dimmesdale's return to his study as his ego retakes possession of his psyche and in a scene of ***anagnorisis*** or recognition, he comes to terms with the moral and psychological consequences of his past and proposed reunion with Hester. This distinctly different man, one with his dignity and self-respect restored, comes to confront his tragic fate and determine the conclusion of the romance.

Each transformation illuminates particular aspects of his evolving psyche and contributes to a more comprehensive understanding of Arthur Dimmesdale and his central place in the inner workings and conclusion of the romance. With its persistent focus on dynamics of the inner life, a psychoanalytically informed understanding of Dimmesdale's psyche can provide a freshly sympathetic perspective on a character who is currently burdened by prevailing negative judgments. I believe that Dimmesdale's character is in need of critical reappraisal. Ullén (2005) notes "the trend over the last three decades in which many critics have been prone to conceive of Dimmesdale's actions in the latter half of the novel in almost entirely negative terms" (p. 119) and further, that:

> To many critics in the fifties, Dimmesdale is the true protagonist of the narrative. From the early seventies onward, however, Dimmesdale's character has been so radically assessed that in some recent readings he seems more of an antagonist of Hester than her beloved (p. 101).

Indeed, contemporary literature critics often express harsh and condemnatory attitudes toward Dimmesdale whose intense and prolonged suffering elicits little compassion. Even so astute and generous a critic as Richard H. Millington (1992) judges that "Dimmesdale exemplifies, in his combination of ambition, narcissism and hunger for endorsement of the authority structure that names him as its own, the tendency of human character to shape itself unthinkingly to the configuration its culture supplies" (p. 85). In contrast, it is Hester's "capacity to love outside the self, to build her life upon her bonds to others that crucially distinguishes her from Dimmesdale" (p. 85). Millington's idealized view of Hester does not take into account that, other than in her attachment to Pearl, she is an isolate who, at a certain point, willfully withdraws from all personal relationships and that Dimmesdale, albeit riddled by guilt, maintains an empathic and loving relationship with his entire congregation. The narrator informs us:

> the Reverend Mr. Dimmesdale had achieved a brilliant popularity in his sacred office. He won it, indeed, in part, by his sorrows.... But this very burden it was, that gave him sympathies so intimate with the sinful brotherhood of mankind; so that his heart vibrated in unison with theirs, and received their pain into itself, and sent its own throb of pain through a thousand other hearts, in gushes of sad, persuasive eloquence (pp. 141–142).

Hester's fortunes in the critical literature have continued to rise in proportion to Dimmesdale's decline. Patricia Dunlavy Valenti's recent essay (2014) represents an extreme example of the trend to debase Dimmesdale. She lauds Hester as "one of the most enduring, iconic figures in American Literature" (p. 33), whereas Dimmesdale is a man whose "impotencies – sexual, emotional, moral, and verbal – infiltrate every area of his life" (p. 24) and, in a conclusion unsubstantiated by the text, she ascribes his progressive deterioration to the sequelae of the practice of "habitual masturbation" (p. 23). In advancing this interpretation, Valenti puts aside the overwhelming textual evidence that the Minister's decline is a consequence of having kept secret the sin of adultery which, as he states at the opening scaffold scene, compels him "to hide a guilty heart through life" (Hawthorne, 1962, Vol. 1, p. 67). Whatever the cultural forces that are at play in shaping her interpretation, it will not do to denigrate Dimmesdale in the service of elevating Hester. Vituperation of Dimmesdale does violence not only to Hawthorne's text but to Hester herself; her devoted attachment to a man anything like this characterization, would show Hester to be iconic, indeed: a two-time loser who knows no better than to return repeatedly to drink from the well of exploitative relationships. The denigration of Dimmesdale and the idealization of Hester collide and undermine each other. As a consequence, the capacity of the two formidable pillars of the romance, Hester Prynne and Arthur Dimmesdale, to bear its profound moral weight is compromised, and the "darkening close of a tale of human frailty and sorrow" (p. 48) becomes depleted of meaning. This is an unfitting prospect for a novel which, in Lawrence Buell's compendious study, *The Dream of the Great American Novel* (2014), is still judged among the most, if not the single most influential work of fiction in the history of American literature. In attempting a more detailed psychological study of Dimmesdale, I hope this chapter will provide an interpretive basis to restore him and his relationship with Hester to the humanely dignified status that they deserve and Hawthorne intended and, *pari passu*, serve in part to stabilize the wide variances in judgments about him.

In his notable essay, "Our Hawthorne" (1964), Lionel Trilling calls attention to how cultural assumptions have had a shaping influence on critical views of Hawthorne. He points out that Henry James' Hawthorne is distinctly different from the tragic Hawthorne of his own era. Gordon Hutner's essay, "Whose Hawthorne" (2004), draws upon Trilling's insights and presents a chilling update to some of his conclusions. Hutner finds that in the intervening fifty years, there has been what amounts to a seismic change in American critical judgments of Hawthorne in that his

> "appeal to the idea of the interiority and the complexity of human motives, his worries about the risks of individualism and the cost of freedom, his skepticism about worldly success, the obdurancy of the material world, all seem…much too irrelevant" (p. 258).

The Hawthorne of today, our Hawthorne, "who sometimes no longer matters at all" is, in Hutner's further assessment of prevailing critical judgments, "an author whose great purpose is to expose his own inauthenticity and debility, thereby unveiling the corruption of the critical world that enshrined him" (p. 258). I would conjecture that the force of recent critical sentiment against Dimmesdale, which focuses so exclusively on his "inauthenticity and debility", is a displacement of culturally determined attitudes toward Hawthorne (p. 258). I agree with Hutner who judges that Hawthorne, "as Trilling evokes him, is a writer, now that his bicentenary has arrived, that we, as a critical era, have lost at our own peril" (p. 258).

If the truth be told, Hawthorne facilitates this transference to Dimmesdale by employing a narrator whose stance toward the minister vacillates unpredictably between irony and empathy. The narrator is a complex character. In The Custom-House, he was drawn to the cloth of the scarlet letter whose "deep meaning" (Vol. 1, p. 31), he admits, "was subtly communicating itself to my sensibilities, but evading analysis of my mind" (p. 31); moreover, its "burning heat" was experienced when "I happened to place it on my breast" (p. 32). The narrator, identifying through his heart with the meaning encoded in the letter, sets his task in writing the tale to imagine "the motives and modes of passion that influenced the characters who figure in it" (p. 33). This imagining finds expression in an empathic voice. We remember, too, the narrator's ironic voice that is prominent throughout The Custom-House, with which he skewers its functionaries, and the government that employs them, as being guilty of hypocrisy, among other things. The narrator does not confine this voice to The Custom-House, as it is distinct in *The Scarlet Letter*, particularly when it speaks of Arthur Dimmesdale.

Critics' skepticism about Hawthorne, articulated by Hutner, finds particular affinity to the narrator's irony toward the minister. In consequence, I speculate, there is a disruption of evenly-hovering critical attention to the equilibrium between the ironic and empathic narratorial voices. A critical reconsideration of Dimmesdale consists in re-establishing this equilibrium by invigorating receptivity to the narrator's empathic voice. We need to place the minister closer to our hearts, and I believe that Hawthorne would have us to do so. Although he strews the road to understanding Dimmesdale with obstacles, he also serves as a guide in this pursuit as he sets out a map, as it were, to reach the goal. In relation to Chillingsworth's attempt to "know" Dimmesdale and discover the secret underlying his illness, the narrator offers the following extraordinarily instructive, cautionary wisdom:

> A man burdened with a secret should especially avoid the intimacy of his physician. If the latter possess native sagacity, and a nameless something more,– let us call it intuition; if he show no intrusive egotism, nor disagreeably prominent characteristics of his own; if he have the power, which must be born with him, to bring his mind into such affinity with his patient's, that this last shall unawares have spoken what he imagines

> himself only to have thought; if such revelations be received without tumult, and acknowledged not so often by an uttered sympathy, as by silence...–then, at some inevitable moment, will the soul of the sufferer be dissolved, and flow forth in a dark, but transparent stream, bringing all its mysteries into the daylight (p. 124).

In this passage Hawthorne presages what Freud, and generations of psychoanalysts who followed him, arrived at concerning the ideal therapeutic relationship between analyst and analysand. In one sweep of the pen, as it were, Hawthorne establishes the theoretical ground for psychoanalytic neutrality, empathic listening, evenly-hovering attention, and attunement to countertransference as crucial parameters in the analytic situation. This study attempts to utilize Hawthorne's guidance to discover "the motives and modes of passion" (p. 33) that influenced his character, Arthur Dimmesdale.

First Transformation: The Office of Guilt

From various comments in the text, one can assemble an extraordinarily impressive portrait of Dimmesdale before his sexual encounter with Hester. He was an Oxford graduate of "scholar-like attainments" (p. 66), "high native gifts" (p. 66) and "eloquence and religious fervor" (p. 66); he was, in essence, a "young and eminently distinguished divine" (p. 238) who had come to the New World as Puritan minister to bring "all the learning of the age into our wild forest-land" (p. 66). Even so critical an observer as Chillingworth finds in the minister "high aspiration for the welfare of his race, warm love of souls, pure sentiments, and natural piety, strengthened by thought and study, and illuminated by revelation" (p.130). Consequently, he was loved, respected and revered by his exacting congregation. This was the man of "invaluable gold" (p. 130) in heart, mind and spirit, that Hester, alone and vulnerable in the community, fell in love with. With her daring imagination, Hester was undoubtedly drawn to this man in whom "thought and imagination were so active, and sensibility so intense" (p. 124). And as a woman who had been ensnared in a passionless marriage with an aging and deformed man, she must have found her Reverend, with his "very striking aspect" (p. 66), a compelling example of vigorous and virtuous manhood. He was the man she once, and after all that transpired, "still so passionately loved (p. 193). And it is his death which defines her as a woman "burdened with a lifelong sorrow" (p. 263). The superlative descriptions of Dimmesdale bely Nina Baym's (1986) judgment that, regarding Hester, "We cannot see in Dimmesdale what she sees in him" and that her love for him was a "delusion...perhaps purely Hester's creation, built from her desire on the sands of Dimmesdale's weaknesses" (p. 26). Hester herself contradicts Baym's assertion. Seeing him on the scaffold during the night vigil, she apprehends the stark contrast between the man before her and the Arthur Dimmesdale she had known: "*Knowing what this poor, fallen man had once been,* her whole soul was moved by the shuddering terror with which he had appealed to her" (p. 159, emphasis added). If we cannot see what Hester saw, perhaps we need to examine our blindness, not hers.

With all his formidable strengths, Dimmesdale's psychological composition was marked with distinctive vulnerabilities. He is described as having a "shy and sensitive reserve" (p. 139) and a highly attuned "nervous sensibility" (p. 66) which were betrayed to the public eye by "an apprehensive, a startled, a half-frightened look" (p. 66). However, something more than acute nervous sensibility is awry in Dimmesdale's psyche as he is "a being who felt himself quite astray and at a loss in the pathway of human existence, and could only be at ease in some seclusion of his own" (p. 66). This description suggests a precarious sense of self in the world. Moreover, the sought-after seclusion that "kept him simple and childlike; coming forth when the occasion was, with a freshness, and fragrance, and dewy purity" (p.66) can be interpreted as an unconscious defense in the service of preventing erotic stimulation and maintaining a regressive sense of innocence and purity. It appears that Dimmesdale, who, in Chillingworth's informed estimation, had inherited "a strong animal nature" (p. 130), had been warding off powerful promptings of *Eros*. With all his "higher, purer, softer qualities" (p. 194), which had carried him to the vertiginous height of his religious profession and community approbation, Dimmesdale also had to contend with "all the violence of passion" (p. 194), deeply repressed, but always under pressure to be expressed and thus to provoke a disastrous fall. Reverend Dimmesdale, alas, is a man like the rest of us. And what will become of him, when trodding in solitude one day on a shadowy by-path, thus attempting to retain a child-like dewy purity of thought, he encounters, on the very same path, his beautiful, "passionate and impulsive" (p. 57) parishioner, Hester Prynne?

Hawthorne provides no details of their sexual liaison. There is much to suggest that Hester and Dimmesdale's encounter in the forest, in the oddly but tellingly named Chapter XVII, "The Pastor and His Parishioner," represents a form of repetition of the encounter which led to their sexual union over seven years before. Each encounter involves physical contact and is followed by a bright but brief glow of newly consecrated love. The repetition is alluded to in the following description after their reunion: "Love, whether newly born, or aroused from a deathlike slumber, must always create a sunshine, filling the heart so full of radiance, that it overflows upon the world" (p. 203).[2] Be that as it may, Dimmesdale knew that Hester was a married woman and that adultery transgresses "one of the most sacred" (p. 200) of received laws. However we imagine their sexual relationship, it comprised a "single instance" (p. 200) which the narrator characterizes, on Dimmesdale's part at least, as "a sin of passion, not of principle, nor even purpose" (p. 200). After the Act came the Word. In the forest, Hester reminds Dimmesdale of what they said after their sexual union. This is the reader's one direct access to the scene: "What we did had a consecration of its own. We felt it so! We said so to each other! Hast thou forgotten it?" Dimmesdale replies, "Hush,

Hester!...No; I have not forgotten!" (p. 195). Hester forces the point that theirs was mutual assent in action, feeling, thought, and interpretation. In the immediate aftermath, their sexual union is imbued with a quality of private consecration.

The fact that Hester is a married woman and pregnant by a man other than her husband and that Dimmesdale is a pastor of a Puritan congregation are inescapable realities which shatter their deep but fragile sentiment of consecration which cannot endure being flung into the public arena with its glaring scrutiny and communal judgments. Their joy is short-lived and their trials are only beginning. We witness Hester's trial on the scaffold in just such a public glare. The source of Dimmesdale's suffering is hidden and thereby uniquely destructive.

Hidden guilt does its inexorable office. By the opening scene of the romance, *in medias res,* Dimmesdale's hitherto healthy self had been transformed, or, rather, deformed by a neurosis and psychosomatic illness of life-threatening severity. That former self was gone. The narrator dispassionately notes, "About this period, however, the health of Mr. Dimmesdale had evidently begun to fail" (p. 120). Given Dimmesdale's psychological vulnerabilities, we can see how the scaffold of shame at the novel's opening represents the perfect storm for his psyche: here Dimmesdale would be thrust out from any refuge afforded by seclusion and subject to the overstimulation of public scrutiny. Hitherto the object of adoration, he would suffer disapprobation, scorn, and rejection which, with Hester and Pearl at his side, would all relate to the exposure, *in flagrante delicto,* of his erotic life. This highlights some of the unconscious aspects of Dimmesdale's fear of exposing his guilty sexuality. On the conscious level, the reality-oriented function of his ego must take into account that public exposure would most likely result, in Chillingworth's words, in being "hurled from the pulpit into a dungeon, - thence, peradventure to the gallows!" (p. 171).[3]

In his exhortation to Hester on the scaffold, Dimmesdale accurately forecasts his fate going forward that if she does not reveal him as her sexual partner: he is destined to "hide a guilty heart through life" and "compel him, as it were - to add hypocrisy to sin" (p. 67). Dimmesdale then admits to Hester what amounts to his tragic flaw, a failure of courage, which prevents him from doing what he asks her to do in his stead: "Take heed how thou deniest him – who, perchance hath not the courage to grasp it for himself–the bitter, but wholesome cup that is now presented to thy lips!" (p. 67). Hester is silent and Dimmesdale survives the scene as an anguished and guilty hypocrite. That the minister appears to be a spotless Puritan clergyman, but is not, constitutes the platform of the narrator's persistent irony toward him which is suffused with condescension and disdain. The minister needs no reminder that he is a hypocrite as he suffers immeasurably from that knowledge: "I have laughed, in bitterness and agony of heart, at the contrast between what I seem and what I am!" (p. 191). Yet, like the fantasied avenging demon in "The Haunted Mind" sketch, the narrator keeps his finger pointed at the minister's hypocrisy, the "sore place in your heart" (Vol. 9, p. 202), and in doing so turns his sympathy, and potentially his reader's, away from his character's profound misery. Arthur Dimmesdale is a man alone in his agony.

Guilt is the secret source of his psychological illness, from which emanates the "poison of one morbid spot…infecting his heart's entire substance" (p. 140). Dimmesdale's psyche is a *locus belli* between the forces of a passionate nature, the id, and the enforcement of a highly developed and punitive superego, further conditioned by the moral rigors of Puritanism. As previously described, Dimmesdale's psyche was already on guard against expressions of libido. The contact with Hester occasioned a flood of erotic energy in which the superego was temporarily incapacitated. This was the sin of passion; Pearl and the scarlet letter are its legacies. In consequence, the *id* has to be further repudiated as the *superego* redoubles its effort at repression with added measures of punishment for the guilty infraction. The *ego*, wedged between the warring agencies of the mind, cannot withstand the onslaught and falls back into a weakened and regressed position. The result is psychological disaster. Moreover, Dimmesdale's diseased mind hastens the progression of a physical ailment for, as Chillingworth tells his patient, there is "A strange sympathy betwixt soul and body!" (p. 138) so that "a sickness, a sore place, if we may so call it, in your spirit hath immediately its appropriate manifestations in your bodily frame" (p. 136). The conflicts arising from guilt are played out in the theatre of Dimmesdale's body.

It was Freud's seminal insight, one that was anticipated by Hawthorne, that repressed instincts continue to push toward gratification, not openly, but in disguised form of neurotic symptoms. Dimmesdale succumbs to a neurosis in which his erotic life survives in the disguised form of obsessions and compulsions. In order to prevent further eruption of sexual wishes, he relentlessly monitors his own mental activities: "Since that wretched epic, *he watched, with morbid zeal and minuteness*, not his acts–, for those it was easy to arrange, – *but each breath of emotion, and his every thought*" (p. 200, emphases added). This obsessional activity is mentally exhausting but fruitless, since, as the narrator rightly concludes, the "enemy," sexual desire, can "force his way again into the citadel" and select "some other avenue" (p. 201). And so it eventually does. The superego will not only monitor urges toward erotic gratification but also punish them. In a miracle of understatement the narrator notes, "His inward troubles drove him to practices" (p. 144); namely, prolonged fasts, sleep-depriving vigils, and sessions of bloody self-flagellation. These compulsions embody the quintessence of masochism. As Freud was to elucidate in *Three Essays on Sexuality,* masochistic rituals are compromise formations in which the libido finds a measure of gratification admixed with pain; the superego is satisfied to inflict the pain. Thus, in private, masochism becomes Dimmesdale's chief form of erotic expression.

In relation to Dimmesdale, Hester all but disappears from the narrative which signals that, as a consequence of guilt, she has been unconsciously relinquished as an object of desire. This is a significant psychological loss since Hester, "so powerful...to sustain" (p. 201), is no longer available to him as an internalized object of support and comfort. Nor can the community interest Dimmesdale to select "some one of the many blooming damsels, spiritually devoted to him, to become his wife...he rejected all suggestions of the kind" (p. 125). All evidence of heterosexual libido disappears from Dimmesdale's consciousness. The irrepressible libido finds other channels for expression: Dimmesdale is unconsciously drawn into an intimate, homoerotic, and regressive relationship with an older man in the person of Chillingworth. As Hester later observes, in utter consternation, "They know each other well, indeed...they have long dwelt together" (p. 235). They become the odd couple: "...the two were lodged in the same house; so that the every ebb and flow of the minister's life-tide might pass under the eye of his anxious and attached physician" (p. 125). Chillingworth's search for the cause of Dimmesdale's illness becomes frankly sadomasochistic: "Roger Chillingworth...strove to go deep into his patient's bosom, delving among his principals, prying into his recollections, and probing everything with a cautious touch, like a treasure-seeker in a dark cavern" (p. 124). One need not be a psychoanalyst to notice that deep delving, probing, and prying into a dark cavern comprise a metaphoric language of sodomy. Chillingworth, gripped by obsessions and compulsions of his own, which serve to exact revenge and torment on his patient, acts as an externalization of Dimmesdale's own punitive superego. He has free access to the Reverend's haunted mind over which he exercises nefarious power: with "a quiet depth of malice" (p. 139) he could "play on him as he chose....and arouse him with a throb of agony...startle him with sudden fear" (p. 140).

It is important to remember that in the face of psychological and physical decline, Dimmesdale continues his exemplary service as pastor to his congregation, the performance of which affords an island of normalcy, or the semblance of it, in a sea of psychological dysfunction. His secret struggle with guilt heightens his "intellectual gifts, his moral perceptions and his power of experiencing and communicating emotion" (p. 141) and increases his empathy with "the sinful brotherhood of mankind" (p. 142). His bond with his congregation is enhanced by his ability to both convey and receive "...pain through a thousand other hearts" (p. 142). Hester's willful silence has, in essence, preserved the minister's ability to serve his community. However much he serves his congregants, his good works bring him no inner peace: "It is inconceivable, the agony with which the public veneration tortured him!" (p. 143). As Dimmesdale predicts in the opening scene, the hypocrisy he feels in his continued functioning as a spiritual leader of the community makes all his substantial contributions to the congregation, and the love and venerations they give rise to, psychologically nugatory. In being but a "remorseful hypocrite" (p. 144) he takes no pleasure in his accomplishments because, "by the constitution of his nature, he loved the truth, and loathed the lie, as few men ever did. Therefore, above all things else, he loathed his miserable self!" (p. 144).

Thus there is no rest for Dimmesdale's psyche, besieged as it is from within and without by a harsh superego determined to exact punishment. By the time of the second scaffold scene, he is on the border of insanity and death. In shock at what she sees at the night vigil, Hester appreciates the depth of Dimmesdale's physical and mental deterioration and discerns Chillingworth's malignant role in his decline: "all her sympathies toward him had been softened and invigorated. She now read his heart more accurately" (p. 193). Dimmesdale's pathetic appeal for her assistance rekindles her love and dedication to his welfare. He is once again "an object that appeared worthy of any exertion and sacrifice for its attainment" (p. 166). As a matter of fact, seven years of trials have also brought Hester to a state of desperation of her own in which she contemplates filicide and suicide as escape from what seems to be an insuperable dilemma of being (p. 166).[4] She finds renewed purpose in her mission to rescue Dimmesdale from Chillingworth's destructive thrall.

Second Transformation: From Melancholia to Mania

Seven years of unrelieved psychological suffering have "shattered and subdued" (p. 197) Dimmesdale's physical and psychological health. Upon his return through the forest from his visit to Apostle Eliot, he is, both in mind and body, *in extremis*, as he "...would have been glad, could he be glad of any thing, to fling himself down at the root of the nearest tree, and lie there passive for evermore" (p. 188). In the ensuing encounter, one that had been carefully calculated by Hester, Dimmesdale begins to revive, literally, with his first touch of her hand. He is indeed rescued from the verge of the darkest abyss by Hester. [5] In response to Dimmesdale's anger at her revelation that Chillingworth is her husband, she throws herself on him in an embrace that, despite his protest, she will not release. Through the power of this embrace, there is a reawakening of their love; memories of their sexual union and its sentiment of consecration are evoked. Hester exhorts Dimmesdale to leave the past behind and forge a new future: "Begin all anew! Hast though exhausted possibility in the failure of this one trial? Not so! The future is yet full of trial and success...Exchange this false life of thine for a true one" (p. 198). She asserts power over Dimmesdale as she is "fixing her deep eyes on the minister's, and instinctively exercising magnetic power over a spirit so shattered and subdued that it could hardly hold itself erect" (p. 197). The language suggests a form of mesmeric influence, certainly not a rational one. Following Hester's assertion "Thou shall not go alone!" (p. 198), Dimmesdale succumbs to the lure of the relief she offers and agrees to elope with her and Pearl to Europe. It is not at all clear that Dimmesdale is persuaded by her arguments which run counter to everything he thinks and believes. What is decisive, and what at the time obscures all other considerations, is the promise of the sustaining comfort of her physical presence which carries with it the quality of psychological salvation "to this poor pilgrim, on his dreary and desert path, faint, sick, miserable, there appeared a glimpse of human affection and a sympathy, a new life, and a true one, in exchange for the one he was now expiating" (p. 200). The narrator abandons irony in this deeply empathic characterization of the minister's plight.

However, in the emotional rush of this scene, the narrator pauses to ask an incisive question: "But Arthur Dimmesdale! Were such a man once more to fall, what pleas could be urged in extenuation of his crime?" (p. 200). Dimmesdale, in an echo of this question, briefly addresses the theological implications of the proposed action with Hester: "O Thou to whom I dare not lift mine eyes, wilt Thou yet pardon me!" (p. 201). Hester's commanding response is concise: "Thou wilt go!" which she says "calmly, as he met her glance" (p. 201). She casts aside a conflict that lies near the core of Dimmesdale's moral being and reasserts the mesmeric influence of her eyes. This will come back to haunt her. Even as Hester and Dimmesdale are joined in a refulgence of this reunion, the narrator stresses that seven years had created an essential psychological and moral chasm between the two of them, one that cannot be bridged "within the magic circle" (p. 200) of but one, solitary hour. Hester "had habituated herself to such a latitude of speculation as was altogether foreign to the clergyman" (p. 199); moreover, "the whole seven years of outlaw and ignominy has been little other than a preparation for this very hour" (p. 200). Dimmesdale, "on the other hand, had never gone through an experience calculated to lead him beyond the scope of generally received laws; although in a single instance, he had so fearfully transgressed one of the most sacred of them" (p. 200). Their sexual union had been a "single instance" of a "sin of passion;" to leave his congregation now, as Hester proposes, with a woman whose husband is alive and now known all too well to him, would be a sin of both principle and purpose. To "Give up this name of Arthur Dimmesdale," as Hester exhorts him to do, "and make thyself another, and a high one, such as thou canst wear without fear or shame" (p. 198) would condemn him, a "man who by the constitution of his nature…loved the truth, and loathed the lie as few men ever did" (p. 144) to another iteration of life as a "remorseful hypocrite" (p. 144).

While in Hester's presence, Dimmesdale experiences the "exhilaration effect – upon a prisoner just escaped from the dungeon of his own heart – of breathing the wild, free atmosphere of an unredeemed, unchristianized, lawless region" (p. 201). Dimmesdale is released, for a time, from the harsh domination of his haunted mind. The "unredeemed, unchristianized and lawless region" is associated with Hester, to whom he has yielded; however, the characterization itself suggests, within the pastor's religious framework, moral regression. The newly found freedom from the constraints of a punitive superego occasions a flood of hitherto repressed libidinal energy. Dimmesdale entered the forest morbidly depressed: "There was a listlessness in his gait; as if he saw no reason for taking one step farther, nor felt any desire to do so" (p. 188). He exits the forest in a highly-charged state: "The excitement of Mr. Dimmesdale's feelings, as he returned from his interview with Hester, lent him unaccustomed physical energy, and hurried him townward at a rapid pace" (p. 216).

From the psychoanalytic perspective, it can be said that Dimmesdale has surrendered the functions of his superego, with its severe self-punitive cast, to Hester's which has been freed from the moorings of Christian moral law: "The world's law was no longer a law for her mind" (p. 164). The mechanism of identifying with the superego of another person or persons is elucidated by Freud (1921) in *Group Psychology and the Analysis of the Ego.* In the same work, Freud describes that the condition of melancholia, characterized by "condemnation of the ego in delusions of inferiority and in self-deprecation," may, if the burden of the superego is relieved, emerge into a state of mania, in which: "the person, in a mood of triumph and self-satisfaction, disturbed by no self-criticism, can enjoy the abolition of his inhibitions, his feelings of consideration for others, and his self-reproaches" (p. 132). I believe that this describes precisely what happens to Dimmesdale: the exhilaration that he feels, and that gives him the experience of unbounded energy, bespeaks the id's new freedom from the constraints of the harsh superego. The depleted psyche is flooded by libidinal energy: "Do I feel joy again?... I seem to have flung myself – sick, sin-stained and sorrow-blackened- down upon these forest-leaves, and to have risen up all made anew" (pp. 201–202).

I want to emphasize, as it is a pillar of upon which my thesis rests, that this release into mania is transient; the superego will soon reassert its powerful position in the psyche and the exhilaration will wane. It is a phenomenon that interested Hawthorne as it is depicted in two other romances. First is the example of Clifford after Jaffrey's death in *The House of the Seven Gables*: "As for us, Hepzibah, we can dance now! – we can sing, laugh, play, do what we will! The weight is gone...off this weary old world; and we may be as light-hearted as little Phoebe herself!" (Vol. 2, p. 250). This state expends itself on the railway journey to nowhere: "He had been startled into manhood and intellectual vigor; or, at least into a condition that resembled them, though it might be both *diseased and transitory*" (Vol. 2, p. 258, emphasis added). Within a short time, the "wild effervescence of his mood...had entirely subsided. A powerful excitement had given him energy and vivacity. Its operation over, he forthwith began to sink" (Vol. 2, p. 266). In a similar vein is the example of Miriam's immediate reaction to Donatello's murder of her nemesis, the Model: "Forget it! Cast it all behind you! ...The deed has done its office, and has no existence anymore" (Vol. 4, p. 176). And so, for a brief time, Miriam and Donatello

> ... flung the past behind them, as she counselled, or else distilled from it a fiery intoxication, which sufficed to carry them triumphantly through of the *first moments* their doom. For, guilt has its *moments* of rapture, too. The foremost result of a broken law is ever an ecstatic sense of freedom (Vol. 4, p. 176, emphases added).

All is not stable in Dimmesdale's psyche as such abrupt and radical mood shifts rarely bode well. Despite his character's exhilaration, Hawthorne soberly titles the chapter, "The Minister in a Maze." With the constraints of the superego temporarily lifted, on his walk home Dimmesdale is flooded with erotic and destructive impulses which he can barely contain. In his encounters on the road he experiences urges "at once involuntary and intentional" (p. 217) to express shocking impieties regarding sacred doctrine and inappropriate erotic suggestions. For instance, in his encounter with a young parishioner, he is tempted to "drop into her tender bosom a germ of evil that would be sure to blossom darkly soon, and bear black fruit, betimes" (pp. 219–220). In *Three Essays on the Theory of Sexuality,* Freud (1905) writes, "A sadist is always at the same time a masochist" (p. 159). It is the subjugation of his superego to Hester's that accounts for his startled experience of a "total change of dynasty and moral code, in that interior kingdom" (p. 217). In Dimmesdale's struggle against the instinctual onslaught, he attempts to locate the inciting agent outside himself: "What is it that haunts me and tempts me thus? Am I mad? Or am I given over to the fiend?" (p. 222). However understandable, the decision to succumb again to what, in his Puritan framework, is a life of sin with Hester has poisoned his moral foundation and awakens in him a potential for "Scorn, bitterness, unprovoked malignity, gratuitous desire for ill and ridicule for whatever was good and holy" (p. 222). In this Walpurgisnacht, the dark vault of Dimmesdale's haunted mind has been flung open and he is forced to encounter the twin fiends of *Eros* and *Thanatos* that dwell therein.

Third Transformation: *Anagnorisis*

As if attempting to flee these fiends, Dimmesdale "hastened up the stairs" and "took refuge in his study" (p. 222). The manic state is extinguished when he re-enters his chamber with its stabilizing appurtenances of his hitherto devout Christian life. As he surveys his familiar surroundings, he recovers his bearings. And when the minister's glance comes upon the Bible, he re-finds, in the moment, his moral compass: "There was the Bible, in its rich old Hebrew, with Moses and the Prophets *speaking to him,* and God's voice through it all!" (p. 223, emphasis added). The dynasty and moral code of the Kingdom of God is re-established in the minister's inner realm; religious devotion there renewed will determine everything he does until his death.

Thus begins Dimmesdale's third transformation. Having achieved a respite from the lashings of the superego and the urgency of the id, Dimmesdale's ego now exercises considerable powers of self-observation, reflection, and integration: "But he seemed to stand apart, and eye this former self with scornful, pitying but half-envious curiosity." These are highly nuanced examples of awareness: scorn involving critical judgment from a superior position, pity requiring sympathetic distance from the object and half-envious curiosity implying the simultaneous operation of an intellectual wish to know intermixed with the regressive wish to return to a state of ignorance. Dimmesdale's intellect and emotions are finally aligned. The nature of this conscious self-reflection allows for a conclusion in which both the narrator and Dimmesdale are conjoined: "That self was gone!" The next statement alludes to the core element of the transformation: "Another man had returned out of the forest; a wiser one; with a knowledge of hidden mysteries which the simplicity of the former never could have reached. A bitter kind of knowledge that!" (p. 223). Surely the Dimmesdale referred to as "another man" is not the one still in the throes of mania, a state of mind inimical to self-reflection and to the acquisition of knowledge and wisdom. The flood of libido has crested and ebbed. No. Dimmesdale is now in a thoughtful and sober mood. The juxtaposition of vastly different moods and rapidly changing states of mind in a short period of time may be confusing, and deliberately so, but unambiguous, at least to a psychoanalyst familiar with tracking such phenomena. Neither oppressed by guilt and depression nor propelled by mania, Dimmesdale is achieving psychic reintegration through painful self-awareness.

In "standing apart," Dimmesdale sees into himself and now knows who his is; there no longer need be a discrepancy between his inner state and outward behavior. The grounds for narratorial irony toward him, his hypocrisy, is now obsolete. However, the narrator continues to beset the minister with ironic insinuation; for example, the injection of the word "seemed" in the phrase, "He seemed to stand apart" injects a hint of doubt about the minister's objectivity during these transformative moments of reflection. When we carefully consider the construction of this statement, "seemed" can be seen to be a narratorial red herring: "scornful, pitying but half-envying curiosity" is so specific in describing a complex state of mind, it is impossible to imagine what the minister might be doing other than what it "seemed." The reader is kept off-balance by this and other ironic inflections, detailed later, until the final scaffold scene, when this veil of irony is finally lifted.[6]

At this juncture, the equilibrium between the empathic and ironic voice is particularly consequential. The *sotto voce* quality of the narrative about Dimmesdale's transformation and the tinge of irony with which the narrator colors it, creates the condition for its being unappreciated. If the reader, lured by irony, misses it, he or she may be in the company of Hawthorne scholars who have concluded that all the minister does subsequently arises from a persistence of the manic state that developed as a consequence of his meeting with Hester. In this light, he is a self-deluded, grandiose, and pathetic figure, or, in Millington's (1992) words, "an unreconstructed narcissist intent on a last dose of celebrity" (p. 94). Amongst this group of critics is Frederick Crews (1996), who, in his psychoanalytic study, comments on these passages but does not take note of the ego's activities of self-observation involved in "standing apart." For him, instead, Dimmesdale's energetic immersion in the composition of the Election Sermon is fueled by the unconscious, a continuation of sexual excitement stimulated by the recent encounter with Hester: "...the Election Sermon is written by the same man who wants to corrupt young girls in the street, and the same newly liberated sexuality" (p. 147).

Nina Baym (1986) does not specifically comment on this passage, but reaches the same conclusion as Crews, namely that Dimmesdale displaces the energy released by his encounter with Hester into the Election Sermon: "With a superhuman effort, he diverts his mad energy to one crowning achievement, and preaches the greatest – and last—sermon of his life" (p. 71). Joel Porte (1969) interprets "Another man had returned out of the forest" to signal that "Now in full contact with his primitive self, Dimmesdale is ready to convert guilt into sexual power" (p. 109). I may be the first to assign the term "manic" to Dimmesdale's state of mind, but these critics' descriptors of him as a "man who wants to corrupt young girls in the street," and who, with "superhuman effort" and "mad energy," is in contact with a sexually driven "primitive self," are all consistent with this designation. The difference lies in what I believe is their failure to appreciate that the state rapidly dissipates, that it was, indeed, "diseased and transitory." Accordingly, they do not appreciate the minister's subsequent powers of self-reflection and conscious integration which are intrinsic to his transformation. Dimmesdale's newly liberated sexuality, esteemed by these critics, shares the same fate as that of Miriam and Donatello's in *The Marble Faun*: "How icy cold is the heart, when the fervour, the wild ecstasy of passion, had faded away, and sunk down among the dead ashes of the fire that blazed so fiercely, and was fed by the very substance of its life!" (Vol. 4, p. 178). Alas, there is not much to celebrate amidst dead ashes.[7]

In another interpretation of the scene, Frederick Newberry (2015) considers Dimmesdale's change in self as regressive rather than progressive: "Back in Boston, enervation accompanied by desuetude restored to normalcy, Dimmesdale will cast aside romantic veneration and satanic impulse in favor of religious devotion, giving up on life in this world for a devoutly assumed life beyond the grave," an action which, in relation to Hester, makes him "finally unworthy of her" (p. 15). Newberry would have the minister follow Hester's command: "Leave this wreck and ruin here where it hath happened! Meddle no more with it! Begin all anew!" (p. 198). Hawthorne's judgment of worth does not accord with Newberry's. By asserting the authority of the minister's ineluctable conscience, Hawthorne makes it clear that is not possible to begin all anew, as the sins of the past must always be reckoned with. Hester will ultimately come to learn this lesson from her pastor.

In a conclusion which runs counter to the current negative trends to which he calls attention, Ullén (2004) insists that Dimmesdale "provides us with an exemplary reaction; a model for us as readers to emulate" (p. 119). He reads the critical passage to indicate that Dimmesdale "has learned, if yet unconsciously, that the whole truth of the scarlet letter must involve spirit and letter alike, that it must accommodate passion and principle, love and law" (p. 120). I do not necessarily disagree with Ullén, but wish to point out that all that he proposes Dimmesdale has learned, in essence a complicated moral and allegorical lesson, would have had to be processed through the highest functions of consciousness and is not unconscious.

Long before any of the critics cited, F.O. Matthiessen, in his monumental *American Renaissance* (1941), interprets Dimmesdale's transformation in the tradition of Greek tragedy in which, in an *anagnorisis*, "the protagonist became aware of the inexorable course of action and his implications in it" (p. 350); moreover, "these crises strike us now as affecting in proportion to their not merely being discoveries of the necessity of external events, but involving also Oedipus's kind of inner, moral recognition" (p. 350). In relation to Dimmesdale's approaching death, Matthiessen concludes: "Such is the crisis that at last brings the wavering minister to confess his guilt and beg for mercy" (p. 350). In his association of Dimmesdale's transformative enlightenment that attends the denouement of Greek tragedy, I find that Matthiessen most accurately captures its essential nature and rightful place in *The Scarlet Letter.* Also in the tragic tradition, the *anagnorisis* propels the hero to unique, definitive action. Indeed, what happens in this scene is the novel's *peripeteia* as it defines the moral trajectory of *The Scarlet Letter* from this point on to its tragic conclusion.

Dismissal of Chillingworth

The moments before Chillingworth intrudes upon him, while he is "occupied with these reflections" (p. 223) do their work decisively, even if, as Hawthorne would have it, silently. In the essay "Puritans and Prigs" (1998), Marilynne Robinson reflects that true morality's "inwardness and quietism makes its presence difficult to sense, let alone quantify" (p. 160). Details of what Dimmesdale thought and felt in his study at this would settle many questions. Instead, the reader is only told that the knowledge Dimmesdale has recently acquired is "bitter," undoubtedly a reference to the consequences of the "infectious poison" of sin that has recently coursed through his moral system. An appreciation of the ways the man has become "a wiser one," the core of the transformation, will be learned by looking at how he resolves the daunting crises he faces.

Dimmesdale's strength is immediately tested as he comes face to face with the man he now knows is his deadly enemy. The first action under the dominion of his transformed self is to resolutely dismiss Chillingworth as his physician, even though there may be serious consequences to his health in the absence of his medical treatments. In face of the fear of death that Chillingworth tries to provoke, Dimmesdale is willing to choose dying over continued subjugation. The regressive symbiosis, with its masochistic surrender, is now severed. For Dimmesdale, a man who had been haunted by cowardice, this is an act of courage. In addition, by encountering the force of his own unconscious erotic and sadistic wishes during his return to his study, they no longer need to be displaced and projected onto the figure of Chillingworth. Dimmesdale has become the sole proprietor of his superego. He can now expel Chillingworth, figuratively and literally, from his psychic landscape. There remains, however, one further action to perform in order to release him from Chillingworth's thralldom forever.

The interchange between Dimmesdale and Chillingworth also offers valuable data as to Dimmesdale's state of mind after he spends time alone in the study. Totally unlike his impulse-ridden behavior in the forest, in his interview with Chillingworth he is cautious, circumspect and dissembling, everything a person who, in Freud's phrase, "enjoy[s] the abolition of his inhibitions" cannot be. Nor can one postulate that Dimmesdale is in mania just before Chillingworth enters, is "sober" with his physician, and then returns to a prior state afterwards. When this "fiery intoxication" is spent, it is permanently so.

Composition of the Election Sermon

Set apart from the influences of both Hester and Chillingworth, Dimmesdale immerses himself in his ecclesiastical mission, a dedication to which determines all he does until his death. He is restored, albeit much changed, to the dignity of The Reverend Master Arthur Dimmesdale that we have not seen heretofore in the romance proper. What the narrator says of him earlier takes on additional force and meaning in the last phase of his life: Dimmesdale was, first and last, "a pure priest, a true religionist, with reverential sentiment largely developed, and an order of mind that impelled itself powerfully along the track of creed, and wore its passage continually deeper with the lapse of time" (p. 123). Indeed, in the brief last few days of his life Dimmesdale reaffirms that for him "it would always be essential to his peace to feel the pressure of faith about him, supporting, while it confined him within its iron framework" (p. 123). Any judgment of Dimmesdale's actions at the end of the romance must take into consideration these enduring characteristics.

Dimmesdale turns immediately to the composition of the Election Sermon and, as he is uniquely attuned to spiritual influences, recognizes that his writing is guided by heavenly inspiration. It emerged "with such an impulsive flow of thought and emotion, that he fancied himself inspired; and only wondered that Heaven should see fit to transmit the grand and solemn music of the oracles through so foul an organ-pipe as he" (p. 225). That Dimmesdale would be the recipient of divine inspiration is foreshadowed by numerous references in the text to the Tongue of Flame, which bestows upon its recipient the capacity of "addressing the whole human brotherhood in the heart's native language" (p. 142). The minister has been readied for this gift over the years by bearing the burden of guilt which "kept him down, on a level with the lowest" and "gave him sympathies so intimate with the sinful brotherhood of mankind" (p. 142). What of the "the grand and solemn music of the oracles" he is audience to in his study are transcribed into the prophetic content of his Election Sermon. In the morning, after having completed the Sermon, the residual mark of divine visitation can be discerned in "the minister's bedazzled eyes" (p. 225).

The narrator injects ironic distance by using the word "fancied" in the phrase "fancied himself inspired." Of course, all inspiration exists in the realm of fancy. It is a device to suggest that Dimmesdale is deluded. However, the next sentence undermines the irony: "he only *wondered* that Heaven should see fit to transmit the grand and solemn music of the oracles through *so foul a pipe as he*" (p. 225, emphases added). This is an act of self-reflection; Dimmesdale is still grounded in himself as a sinning and defective person and cannot understand why he has been an instrument of divine pronouncement. He is humble in the face of election. A person suffering from delusion and in "a mood of triumph and self-satisfaction, disturbed by no self-criticism" that Freud describes, would consider himself wonderfully deserving to be a divine instrument or that he is divinity, Himself.[8]

The Minister Alone: The Shadow of Death

The reader loses sight of Dimmesdale after this brief view of him in the morning until he reappears, two days later, in the Election procession toward the Meeting House. Dimmesdale's inner workings during this interval would be of considerable interest to the reader. However, in keeping with the sentiment articulated in the The Custom-House introduction, at this time of utmost significance, Hawthorne silences the narrator and thus keeps Dimmesdale's "inmost Me behind its veil" (p. 4). There will be no repetition of voyeuristic violation of the sanctity of his human heart that he had been subjected to for so long.

The pastor has matters of great significance to consider. After all, he has left Hester at the verge of the forest with the agreement to leave everything behind and sail away with her and Pearl immediately after Election Day. In the brief span of time since he left them there has been a dizzying convergence of circumstance: a fearful rush of sexual energy and sinful impulse on the walk home, an *anagnorisis* in the study, the dismissal of Chillingworth, and a dazzling visitation of heavenly inspiration for the Election Sermon. None of these is known to Hester, which helps account for her disorientation and misapprehension of the minister during the Election Day procession: "How deeply they had known each other then! And was this the man? She hardly knew him now!" (p. 239). What both Hester and the reader do not yet know, and will not know until the third scaffold scene, is the circumstance of utmost significance: Dimmesdale, in this interval, comes to the realization that he is "a dying man" (p. 254). Everything to be considered, everything to be decided upon and all that follows in the romance must be understood in the light of this awareness of imminent death. For a spiritual, intelligent, and sensitive person, such as Dimmesdale, we need only imagine the nature of the meditations in which he attempts to reconcile, as a dying man must, all his past and present experience, and comes to decide how he will conduct the brief remainder of his life. It is a true test of the man he was and the man he became. This is, of course, the subject of tragedy. Even though we do not know these reflections, we do know that they propel him to two final actions: the delivery of the divinely inspired Election Sermon and a public confession of sin on the scaffold of shame.

The Election Sermon: The Tongue of Flame

Although widely respected for his outstanding and persuasive oratory, the Election Sermon is Arthur Dimmesdale's *magnum opus.* The reader does not have access to its words, but its unique prosody is refracted through Hester's consciousness as she stands outside the Meeting Hall. It is a remarkably deep and intimate interchange between the congregation and its minister. In its various strains are conveyed expressions of "the suffering of humanity, that touched the sensibility in every bosom!" (p. 243). Anticipating the revelation on the scaffold and expressed in the second language of the heart, Dimmesdale's oration is suffused with the sentiment of the pain "of a human heart, sorrow-laden, perchance guilty, telling its secret, whether of guilt or sorrow, to the great heart of mankind; beseeching its sympathy or forgiveness, - at every moment, - in each accent, – and never in vain!" (p. 243–244). The years of good works and dedication to his community are rewarded with its loving acceptance and forgiveness of his flawed nature. The content of Dimmesdale's oratory fulfills its prophetic intent: "...toward the close, a spirit as of prophecy had come upon him...it was his mission to foretell a high and glorious destiny for the newly gathered people of the Lord" (p. 249). The message could not have been more exigent nor uplifting to the Puritan community whose guiding purpose was to establish a New Jerusalem as God's heavenly dominion on earth. Depth and potency to the prophetic message are added by its being the utterance of a dying man: "through the whole discourse, there had been a certain deep, sad undertone of pathos, which could not be interpreted otherwise than as the natural regret of one soon to pass away" (p. 249). The minister's oratory reaches toward a transfiguration or heavenly apotheosis:

> The idea of his transitory stay on earth gave the last emphasis to the effect which the preacher had produced; it was as if an angel, in his passage to the skies, had shaken his bright wings over the people for an instant, –at once a shadow and a splendor, –and had shed down a shower of golden truths upon them (p. 249).

Lest there be any doubt as to the rectitude of Dimmesdale's final adherence to what he deeply believes to be God's Law, everything in the narration of this scene suggest that, in his piety and humility, he has been visited by a Tongue of Flame, or something like it, as "the last and rarest attestation of his office" (p. 142).[9] The prophetic tradition of Western Christianity, as it inhabits the textual world of *The Scarlet Letter,* stands in support of Dimmesdale's final actions. Dimmesdale, "a pure priest, a true religionist," remains faithful to his innermost self and his sacred calling.

The Revelation of the Scarlet Letter: Tragic Apotheosis

With the mission of the Sermon accomplished, the spiritual energies that invested him wane quickly.[10] Consequently, Dimmesdale struggles to muster sufficient energy to get to the scaffold. It is clear from this that his surfeit of energy was a heavenly investment only for the purpose of delivering a prophetic message. The confession has to be derived from his own strength of will. In an interval of two days Dimmesdale decides, as to what would be his last mortal act, to do what he had not been able to do seven years before: mount the scaffold with Hester and Pearl and confess his partnership in sin. Whereas, it was "Cowardice which invariably drew him back" (p. 148) from public confession, he now, in an undoing of his failure at the opening of the romance, finds "the courage to grasp it for himself" (p. 67).

Continued submission to Chillingworth or fleeing the community were the only alternatives considered by Hester. Given what she accurately perceived as his broken state, Hester was understandably prone to misgauge Dimmesdale's potential. Chillingworth, counting on Dimmesdale's subjugation to the threat of exposure, also underestimates him. The narrator gives no hint of a creative third alternative, confession, that Dimmesdale arrives at. Only Hawthorne knows of his heroic potential and keeps it, as the surprise ending to the romance, hidden from the reader until it is revealed in a moment of extraordinary emotional and moral power.

As he feels his life coming to an end, Dimmesdale, with an elemental Puritan belief in an eternal afterlife, needs to prepare and purify his soul for the next world. He has compounded the sin of adultery with the hypocrisy of silence, both need to be repented through public confession. And so he does. Nor is it easy. There is no injection of manic energy to bolster him for this solemn task. He struggles against inner resistances to face the dreaded public self-exposure. In this he calls upon Hester's support. However, he makes it clear to Hester that he will be assisted by her strength but, in what may be an allusion to his revelation, guided by "the will which God hath granted me!" (p. 253). Dimmesdale will no longer be led by Hester's will, as may have been true in the past, but only by God's.

In the only reference to their recent encounter in the forest, he confronts Hester with the question: "Is this not better… than what we dreamed of in the forest?" (p. 254). And in an allusion to her fantasies of filicide and suicide, Hester responds: "I know not! I know not!…Better? Yea; so we may both die and little Pearl with us!" (p. 254). Hester is angry with Dimmesdale since he has apparently reneged on their agreement. She is not aware of all that transpired in him since they parted. He hastens to impart to her the missing crucial information: "For, Hester, I am a dying man" (p. 254). Bringing her and Pearl to the scaffold with him is, in essence, a final act of love and affirmation of their familial bond as well as a statement about his sexuality and procreativity. It also indicates to Pearl and the community that she is his daughter. Hester is finally acknowledged as his partner and beloved. No longer obscure outcasts, both are elevated by their intimate association with the Reverend; because of this, their position in the mind of the community undoubtedly will never be the same. Dimmesdale's last words to Hester are as pastor to parishioner. In a response to her threat of self-destructive action, he reminds her that her fate is in God's hands not her own. As Hester now knows that he is on the verge of death, perhaps viewing eternity, she turns to him as a guide and seer to ask him what he envisions for their future together. Dimmesdale replies that he cannot see into this but he knows that they have broken God's law. He issues a final theological judgment against the enchantment in the forest: their act had been a violation, not a consecration, of their souls. As to her future, Dimmesdale instructs Hester to think only of their sin, a corrective for her tendency to lawless speculation and action. His last act is to address Pearl and receive her long-awaited kiss. With an invocation to God, he dies.

In judging Dimmesdale's final acts, it is important to remember what actually are his options. The two brief revivals of energy, profane and sacred, occasioned both by the reunion with Hester and divine illumination have passed. Chillingworth's pharmacologic treatments have been withdrawn and death is imminent. As it relates to his sin, Dimmesdale can choose to die unobtrusively with his secret undisclosed or, do what he does, as an act of penitence, confess his partnership in sin with Hester. Dying without disclosure would do little else than preserve his publicly spotless reputation to all but Hester and Chillingworth. Fleeing with Hester and Pearl was no longer a consideration; the escape plot was devised in the charm of the forest, apart from hard realities of encroaching mortality. In any case, there is no escaping Chillingworth who has already arranged to accompany them to Bristol. Dimmesdale knows only too well that freedom from him would come only on the scaffold.

In seeing deeply into his own flawed nature, in facing the inevitability of his fate, and, within the narrowest constraints of time and opportunity, courageously taking the difficult path toward redemption, Dimmesdale achieves the status of tragic hero. Matthiessen (1941) specifies him as one of Hawthorne's protagonists, who, in the tradition of Greek tragedy, "finally face their evil and know it deserving of the sternest justice, and thus participate in the purgatorial movement, the movement toward regeneration" (p. 350). Dimmesdale's final transformation readies him for this movement. Like the Chorus at the conclusion of Greek tragedy, the community reacts to Dimmesdale's death scene with the signature catharsis: "the great heart" of the people "…was thoroughly appalled, yet overflowing with tearful sympathy, as knowing that some deep life-matter – which, if full of sin, was full of anguish and repentance likewise – was now to be laid open to them" (p. 254). And immediately after Dimmesdale dies, "[t]he multitude, silent till then, broke out in a strange, deep voice of awe and wonder, which could not as yet find utterance, save in this murmur that rolled so heavily after the departed spirit" (p. 257).

The reader, one of the multitude, needs to look into his or her own heart to assess the personal impact of Dimmesdale's scene of death. The narrative structure builds in tensions and ambivalences with regard to it. The narrator makes sure that we are not prepared for it and, like Hester, we are disoriented by it. To the extent we are sympathetic to the extreme and protracted suffering of the protagonists and fervently wish for their release in a new and happy life together far away from claustrophobic, Puritan Boston, we are significantly disappointed by it. And to the degree that Hester has won our hearts, we share her anger and rebellion against it.

Hawthorne's art, expressed in the transcendent beauty of the narration of the scene, brings us around to accept the inevitability of the tragic outcome. The narrator of The Custom-House, who felt the burning heat of the scarlet letter when he applied it to his heart, employs no distancing tone of irony here. I agree completely with Ullén's (2004) judgment of the scene's power:

> Whatever we may think of Dimmesdale's 'triumphant' revelation, it can hardly be denied that it is depicted as possessing no small amount of grandeur by the narrator....I would instruct the reader who remains skeptical on this point to try reading the passage aloud – which is, after all, the way Hawthorne read it to Sophia: it is impossible not to be taken in by Dimmesdale's plight in this scene through the sheer pathos of the narrator's tone, echoing that of Dimmesdale himself (p. 384).

Ullén insightfully appreciates that Hawthorne imposes on his reader the responsibility to traverse the distance created by the narrative's irony to arrive at an empathic immersion in the scene's tragic pathos. We will then have arrived, finally, at the "inevitable moment" when "the soul of the sufferer [will] be dissolved, and flow forth in a dark, but transparent stream, bringing all its mysteries into the daylight"(Hawthorne, 1962, Vol. 1, p. 124). Hawthorne's own emotional reactions to the scene are instructive; years later he reports that while reading the last chapters to Sophia his voice had "swelled and heaved, as if I were tossed up and down on an ocean as it subsides after a storm" (Mellow, 1980, p. 311).

One of the profound purposes of tragedy, concerning "deep life-matters" as it does, is to inform the moral life of those who witness it. Dimmesdale's final transformation brings him to choose confession on the scaffold as the site of his death. The consequences of the scene of Dimmesdale's death are felt in the consequent moral transformations, all redemptive, in those who stood nearest to him at the scaffold: Pearl, Chillingworth, and Hester. With the kiss Pearl bestows upon Dimmesdale, "[a] spell was broken" (p. 256) and her vexing search for her father is ended. The ineffable sadness of losing her father at the moment she finds him brings tears that "were the pledge she would grow up amid human joy and sorrow, not for ever do battle with the world, but be a woman in it" (p. 256). There is reason to believe that Chillingworth, before his death, seeks a path of forgiveness and repentance by bequeathing upon Pearl the entirely of his substantial fortune, bringing new meaning to what he had said to Hester in prison: "Thou and thine, Hester Prynne, belong to me" (p. 76). In doing this, he is heeding the spiritual urgency of the minister's last words to him: "May God forgive thee! Thou, too hast deeply sinned!" (p. 256).

In the course of a few moments, Hester has lost, forever, the man she loves. As if she received a blow to the head, she is stunned into silence. We hear only that not long after Chillingworth's death, "the wearer of the scarlet letter disappeared, and Pearl with her" (p. 261). Hester's measured and profound reply to the scene of Dimmesdale's death, spanning years in its formulation but only paragraphs in the text, is encoded in her return, as a transformed woman, to Boston. As a "sad and lonely mother" (p. 262) who is "burdened with a life long sorrow" (p. 263), there is the work of mourning still to be done, which, according to the logic of the romance, can uniquely be accomplished around the site of the scaffold, where "her whole orb of life, before and after, was connected with this spot, as with the one point that gave it unity" (p. 244). Hester returns to Boston to bring herself to unity, psychologically, morally, and spiritually. In this endeavor, Arthur Dimmesdale is her guide. By reassuming the scarlet letter as an exertion of "her own free will" (p. 263), she is following Dimmesdale's last words of instruction to her: "The law we broke! – the sin here so awfully revealed! Let these alone be in thy thoughts!" (p. 256). Like Dimmesdale before her, she transmutes the spectacle of penance into the attitude and acts of repentance and, as a member of the community, she dedicates her life to unique service as a wonderful counselor to the welfare of her "flock". In doing so, she "gained from many people the reverence due to an angel" (p. 32).

Hester's return to Boston constitutes, in its unique way, a definitive judgment of Arthur Dimmesdale. She is not party to the influences of the narrator's irony toward him. She knew him intimately and was witness to his final words and action. To the degree we respect and honor Hester, we should be guided in our appreciation of him by her loyalty to him and to his memory. She follows the path inspired by Dimmesdale to her grave, which the community, in its generosity of spirit, situates next to his. That they are united, but only in death, constitutes the essence of their tragic destiny. And the transformations which inhere in their separate return to the traumatic site of the scaffold are best expressed in the language of poetry, not psychology, as in T.S. Eliot's *The Four Quartets*: "we shall not cease from exploring/ And the end of all our exploration/ Will be to arrive where we started/ And know the place for the first time."[11]

Notes

1. The narrator of the sketch awakens after midnight and describes his mind as being in "an intermediate zone where the business of life does not intrude" (Vol. 9, p. 305); in this state he is the recipient of "Passion and Feeling" which are experienced viscerally or "may assume bodily shape, and things of the mind become dim spectres of the eye" (p. 306). We can reword this description in the language of psychoanalysis as follows: between sleep and wakefulness, the ego's defensive operations are suspended and the psyche becomes the stage for expressions of the id in opposition to the forces of the superego. This conflict of desire and conscience is condensed, in Hawthorne's imagination, into visual, personified images. It is here that Hawthorne's psychology and proclivity toward allegory intersect.
2. Hawthorne anticipates Freud's concept of the repetition compulsion, developed in *Beyond the Pleasure Principle*, which concerns the proclivity of the psyche to re-enact deeply conflicted or traumatic events. In *The Scarlet Letter* the narrator expresses this is relation to the scaffold, but, I believe, it is as true of the forest scene: "But there is a fatality, a feeling so irresistible that it has the force of doom, which almost invariably compels human being to linger around and haunt, ghost- like, the spot where some great and marked event has given the color to their lifetime" (pp. 79–80).
3. Hester later poignantly explains her silence at the scaffold as well as her acquiescence to Chillingworth's oath of silence that he was her husband in the following statement to Dimmesdale: "Truth was the one virtue which I might have held fast, and did hold fast through all extremity;...save when thy good, -thy life, -thy fame were put in question!" (p. 193). She is mindful of the severe punishment that would await her partner in sin. Moreover, pointing the finger of guilt at Dimmesdale would not have lessened her punishment as an adultress; if anything, perhaps because she could be accused of being an agent of Satan who seduced a holy man, it would have been considerably more severe.
4. The narrator writes of Hester: "...a fearful doubt strove to possess her soul whether, it were not better to send Pearl at once to heaven, and go herself to such futurity as Eternal Justice would provide" (p. 166).
5. Of similar nature in the transformation wrought in the despairing and distraught narrator of "The Haunted Mind" when he has a fantasy of a woman lying next to him in his bed. Holgrave, also, is transformed by Phoebe's reappearance at the end of *The House of the Seven Gables:* "The world looked strange, wild, evil, hostile...But, Phoebe, you crossed the threshold; and hope, warmth and joy came in with you!" (Vol. 2, p. 306).
6. Moreover, if the minister is still a hypocrite and is only seeming to look at himself objectively, why would the narrator exclaim, "The self was gone!" and what can be the knowledge and wisdom with which he returned from the forest? A Hawthorne scholar, who generously read an earlier version of this essay, was unconvinced that any transformation had, in fact, taken place because of the doubt introduced in his mind by the word "seemed". It is for this reason, I have attempted to deconstruct it in its context. It is breathtaking that Hawthorne fashioned his text with an exquisite precision that permits such interpretive range regarding the same passage. One word, "seemed", can send interpreters in widely different directions.
7. The appearance of a religious re-awakening so soon after a renewal of sexual energies invites speculation as to their relationship. The critics cited here interpret them as unconsciously flowing from one to the other. As I have tried to demonstrate, the sexual energies that drove Dimmesdale on

his return home have dissipated and are further arrested by the renewed executive functions of his ego. The minister is now in a position to account for the evil that urgent sexuality had brought with it: "Scorn, bitterness, unprovoked malignity, gratuitous desire for ill and ridicule for whatever was good and holy" (p. 222). With his acute moral sensibility, one would imagine that he is aghast. In this light, Dimmesdale's religious re-dedication serves, among other things, as a repudiation of the sexual instincts so recently reawakened. I think that this may be what he is referring to when, in the final scene, he says to Hester: "Is not this better...than what we dreamed of in the forest?" (p. 254). I do not conceptualize his religious fervor as having had its source in sexual instinct which was then used for transcendent purpose; I believe it flowed from a different origin. Freud was reductionistic when it came to spirituality. Many mysteries still surround the ground where even angels fear to tread.

8. Another ironic lure is offered in the second scaffold scene when the narrator intimates that Dimmesdale's singular vision of an immense red letter A in the sky during his night vigil is probably "a symptom of a highly disordered mental state", and that he had "extended his egotism over the entire expanse of nature" (p. 155). However, at the end of the chapter we are told that the same sign was seen by others in the community. The narrator, who has proven himself unreliable, seems unaware that this contradicts his insinuation that this vision is a product of Dimmesdale's mental derangement.
9. The narrator remarks that Dimmesdale's sermon had converted the atmosphere of the church "into words of flame" (p. 248).
10. The narrator insinuates that Dimmesdale may be basking in the glory of the reception to his Sermon at Hester's expense: "He stood, at this moment, on the very proudest eminence of superiority, to which the gifts of intellect, rich lore, prevailing eloquence, and a reputation of whitest sanctity, could exalt a clergyman in New England's earliest days..." (p. 249). The contrast with Hester's position as then described could not be more stark: "Meanwhile, Hester Prynne was standing beside the scaffold of the pillory with the scarlet letter still burning on her breast!" (p. 250). We are led to feel the injustice of Dimmesdale's elevation and Hester's debasement. The irony is, of course, that Dimmesdale knows that he is about to die facing his shame and does not participate in this supposed elevation. Instead, in a few minutes, he will call upon Hester's physical assistance to mount the scaffold without whose strength he declares he would be "groveling down upon my face!" (p. 254).
11. *T.S. Eliot: The Complete Poems and Plays*. Harcourt, Brace and Co. (New York), 1934, p. 145.

References

Baym, N. (1986). *The Scarlet Letter: A Reading*. Boston: Twayne Publishers.

Buell, L. (2014). *The Dream of the Great American Novel*. Cambridge: Harvard University Press.

Crews, F. (1996). *The Sins of the Father: Hawthorne's Psychological Themes*. New York: Oxford University Press.

Eliot, T. S. (1934). *The Complete Poems and Plays*. New York: Harcourt, Brace and Co.

Freud, S. (1905). Three Essays on the Theory of Sexuality. In J. Strachey, A. Freud, A. Strachey, & A. Tyson, (Trans.), *Standard Edition* ((Vol. 7, pp. 123–246). London: Hogarth.

Freud, S. (1920). Beyond the Pleasure Principle. In J. Strachey, A. Freud, A. Strachey, & A. Tyson, (Trans.), *Standard Edition*. (Vol. 7, pp. 65–134) London: Hogarth.

Freud, S. (1921). Group Psychology and the Analysis of the Ego. In J. Strachey, A. Freud, A. Strachey, & A. Tyson, (Trans.), *Standard Edition* (Vol. 18, pp. 65–134). London: Hogarth.

Hawthorne, N. (1962a). *The House of the Seven Gables*. In W. Charvat (Ed.), *The Centenary Editions of the Works of Nathaniel Hawthorne* (Vol.2). Columbus: Ohio University State Press.

Hawthorne, N. (1962b). *The Marble Faun*. In W. Charvat (Ed.), *The Centenary Editions of the Works of Nathaniel Hawthorne* (Vol.4). Columbus: Ohio State University Press.

Hawthorne, N. (1962c). *The Scarlet Letter*. In W. Charvat (Ed.), *The Centenary Editions of the Works of Nathaniel Hawthorne* (Vol.1). Columbus: Ohio State University Press.

Hawthorne, N. (1974). The Haunted Mind. In W. Charvat (Ed.), *The Centenary Editions of the Works of Nathaniel Hawthorne* (Vol.9). Columbus: Ohio University State Press.

Hutner, G. (2004). Whose Hawthorne. In R. H. Millington (Ed.), *The Cambridge Companion to Nathaniel Hawthorne*. Cambride: Cambridge University Press.

Keegan, P. (2017). From Shtetl to Boulevard. *The London Review of Books*, *39*.

Matthiessen, F. O. (1941). *American Renaissance: Art and Expression in the Age of Emerson and Whitman*. New York: Oxford University Press.

Mellow, J. (1980). *Nathaniel Hawthorne and His Times*. Baltimore and London: The Johns Hopkins University Press.

Millington, R. H. (1992). *Practicing Romance: Narrative Form and Cultural Engagement in Hawthorne's Fiction*. Princeton: Princeton University Press.

Newberry, F. (2015). Hawthorne by the Way. *Nathaniel Hawthorne Review*, *40*.

Porte, J. (1969). *The Romance in America: Studies in Cooper, Poe, Hawthorne, Melville and James*. Middletown, CT: Wesleyan University Press.

Robinson, M. (1998). Puritans and Prigs. In *The Death of Adam*. Boston: Houton Mifflin.

Trilling, L. (1964). Our Hawthorne. In R. H. Pearce (Ed.), *Hawthorne Centenary Essays*. Columbus, Ohio: Ohio State University Press.

Ullén, M. (2004). *The Half-Vanished Structure: Hawthorne's Allegorical Dialectics*. Bern: Peter Lang.

Valenti, P. D. (2014). 'Then, all was spoken!' What 'The Custom-House' and *The Scarlet Letter* Disclose. *Nathaniel Hawthorne Review*, *40*.

3 Holgrave's Transformation in *The House of the Seven Gables*: "The black moment became at once a blissful one"

With Jaffrey Pyncheon's death and the flight of Clifford and Hepzibah, *The House of the Seven Gables* (Hawthorne, 1962) reaches its long-anticipated denouement. Destruction is once again visited upon the Pyncheons with a force whose inevitability is akin to what Freud would later characterize as the repetition compulsion. Like his uncle three decades earlier, Jaffrey Pyncheon is overtaken by fatal apoplexy, and Clifford, after thirty years of imprisonment for a crime he did not commit, is once again implicated in the death of a Pyncheon. Earlier in the novel, Holgrave forecasts a crisis to Phoebe: "There is a conviction in me that the end draws nigh" (p. 217), and in an apt theatrical metaphor, he senses "that Destiny is arranging its fifth act for a catastrophe" (p. 218). He also intuits that Jaffrey and Clifford are the principals in the impending confrontation: "Judge Pyncheon! Clifford! What a complex riddle—a complexity of complexities—do they represent!" (p. 179). Holgrave's involvement in this crisis, so he believes, is solely intellectual: "to look on, to analyze, to explain matters to myself, and comprehend the drama which, for almost two hundred years, has been dragging its slow length over the ground, where you and I now tread" (p. 216). In this drama, he anticipates his role to be that of a detached observer: "Providence ... sends me only as a privileged and meet spectator" (p. 217). The reality turns out to be quite contrary to this expectation; when the catastrophe indeed strikes, Holgrave's discovery of Jaffrey's corpse catalyzes a painful and momentous psychological transformation:

> Could you but know, Phoebe, how it was with me, the hour before you came! ... A dark, cold, miserable hour! The presence of yonder dead man threw a great black shadow over everything; he made the universe, so far as my perception could reach, a scene of guilt, and of retribution more dreadful than guilt. The sense of it took away my youth. I never hoped to feel young again! The world looked strange, wild, evil, hostile; —my past life so lonesome and dreary; my future, a shapeless gloom, which I must mould into gloomy shapes! (p. 306)

Holgrave, hitherto so cool and detached, is describing a psychological implosion characterized by a pervasive depression, alienation, and despair. The young man about whom the narrator has vaunted that "amid all these personal vicissitudes, he had never lost his identity," (p. 177) comes perilously close to psychological decompensation in witnessing this scene. No less dramatic is the next turn of his mind in which he says to Phoebe:

> But, Phoebe, you crossed the threshold; and hope, warmth, and joy, came in with you! The black moment became at once a blissful one. It must not pass without the spoken word. I love you! (p. 306)

Following this avowal, and within the precinct of these moments of tender affection, Holgrave has a presentiment, which is soon borne out, that his radicalism will soften into social conformity and that his stance against the hereditary rights of property will yield to his establishing a permanent home with Phoebe in whom resides his "only possibility of happiness" (p. 306) and whose "poise will be more powerful than any oscillating tendency of mine" (p. 307).

Indeed, in the course of a single hour, Holgrave's "oscillating tendency" is expressed in his traversing the wide distance not only from despair to bliss but also from detached spectator to engaged participant, from inveterately independent to openly dependent young man, and from social radical to conservative.[1] These antitheses indicate not just a marked change of mood but a far-reaching psychological transformation of enduring moment. What has been referred to by Rudolphe Von Abele (1955) as Holgrave's "conversion" of social philosophy has received much critical attention (p. 59); the psychological transformation from which it immediately arises has not been the subject of scholarly analysis. It is the purpose of this essay to address that deficiency. Nina Baym's (1970) commentary on this scene is not atypical of the prevailing contemporary critical judgments: "Something goes wrong between the time he enters the parlor … and the time of Phoebe's return. Holgrave undergoes a striking change in character. His social radicalism is gone; he is prepared to abandon his art and take over the routines of a country squire. Instead of finding himself in the darkened parlor, he loses himself" (pp. 593–594). This study is an exploration of "something goes wrong" and arrives at a very different judgment. By looking systematically at the psychological processes that underlie the change in his radical social philosophy, I will conclude that, in the darkened parlor, Holgrave does not lose, but, indeed, finds himself.

What is the psychology of this transformation? More specifically, how can its suddenness, intensity, and pervasive disorientation be accounted for based on what we have come to know of the young Holgrave's psychology? Why is this all precipitated by Jaffrey Pyncheon's dead body? Finally, why does Phoebe's appearance transmute this black moment into a blissful one and then serve to promote a change in Holgrave's social philosophy? These crucial questions have not, to my knowledge, been systematically posed; they will be approached from the perspective of psychoanalytic psychology, which privileges an understanding of the dynamic interweaving of the conscious and unconscious mind that is inevitably at play in a psychological change of this magnitude. The answers, I contend, not only have a significant bearing on a fresh understanding of Holgrave's fate but also provide the context to better understand aspects of the novel's much-disputed "happy ending."

A psychoanalytic framework in the tradition of Freud was largely prefigured by Hawthorne, and thus his texts are congenial to Freudian analysis. The prototype for the system of psychology that informs *The House of the Seven Gables* (1851) was put forth with succinctness and force in Hawthorne's early sketch "The Haunted Mind" (1835), which anticipates, with uncanny accuracy, Freud's topographic model of the mind in its delineation of the terrain of id, ego, and superego and the forces that govern their interaction. The psychological trials of the narrator in "The Haunted Mind" look forward to those of Holgrave with remarkable exactitude, indicating a stability of Hawthorne's psychological insights over time. Both the sketch's narrator and Holgrave, finding themselves alone and in vulnerable states of mind, are possessed by images of death and are haunted by the dark associations to which they give rise; both are rescued from their torments by the appearance of a loving woman. Magisterially, the narrator of "The Haunted Mind" generalizes about the precise nature of the psyche: "In the depth of every heart, there is a tomb and a dungeon, though the lights, the music, and the revelry above, may cause us to forget their existence, and the buried ones, or prisoners whom they hide. But sometimes, and oftenest at midnight, those dark receptacles are flung wide open" (Vol. 9, p. 306). For both Hawthorne and Freud, the unconscious is a dynamic force that always presses upward toward expression; stored as unconscious, affect-laden memory, the past forever haunts the present. At certain crucial times, the contents of the haunted mind may flood into consciousness and produce far-reaching disruption of psychic functioning. Such a confrontation with the repressed is precisely what Holgrave experiences in his hour-long vigil with Jaffrey Pyncheon's corpse and is a precondition for the transformation that follows.

Holgrave's "ghosts and prisoners," which haunt his unconscious and are released during the fateful hour, are related to his secret: he is a Maule, who, despite his hitherto-peripatetic existence, has taken up residence in the House of the Seven Gables and is its present-day nemesis. He professes to Phoebe that he will "dwell in it for a while, that I may know the better how to hate it" (Vol. 2, p. 184). This hatred is the living legacy of the Maules' aggressive wishes for revenge against the Pyncheons. That he is a Maule is revealed to Phoebe and to the reader at the end of the novel: "My dearest Phoebe … how will it please you to assume the name of Maule? … You should have known sooner, (only I was afraid of frightening you away,) that, in this long drama of wrong and retribution, I represent the old wizard, and am probably as much of a wizard as he ever was" (p. 316). This confession, coming near the end of the story, leads us to re-index all that we know of him in the light of this revelation and to construct a revised narrative about him that includes this crucial, hidden fact of his history.

This is not the first application of a psychoanalytic lens to Holgrave's mental crisis. In the widely cited psychoanalytic study of Hawthorne's fiction, *The Sins of the Father*, Frederick Crews (1966) is alert to this marked change in Holgrave that occurs in this scene: "Without apparent reason, the resourceful and independent daguerreotypist is oppressed by the figure of Jaffrey Pyncheon in death" (p. 188). Crews observes that, although "Holgrave's fear of 'retribution' has no basis in stated motive, yet it reminds us that his view of society and history has been metaphorically Oedipal" and offers the interpretation that "Jaffrey's death thus satisfies a patricidal strain in Holgrave's nature—a fact which is corroborated by his 'unmotivated' anxiety before Jaffrey's corpse" (p. 188). There is much, that is, unsatisfying in Crews's interpretation. It overlooks the fact that the guilt and retribution that Holgrave reads into this scene belong, first and foremost, to Jaffrey Pyncheon, whose crime against Clifford, of which Holgrave had knowledge, resulted in his cousin's long imprisonment; the possible links between Jaffrey's guilty crime and what Crews posits as Holgrave's fear of retribution are never advanced. Moreover, in ascribing Holgrave's anxiety to the workings of a "metaphoric" Oedipal conflict that is projected onto the paternal figure of Jaffrey, Crews fails to take into account the actual, as distinct from the symbolic, nature of Holgrave's relationship to Jaffrey. Holgrave knew Jaffrey Pyncheon all too well; the Judge had been his client in whose daguerreotype portrait the artist revealed his pernicious character, which hid cruelty and avarice under a facade of benevolence. He professes to Phoebe: "Here we have the man, sly, subtle, hard, imperious, and, withal, cold as ice. Look at that eye! Would you like to be at its mercy?" (Hawthorne, 1962, Vol. 2, p. 92). Finally, Crews's interpretation does not consider the long history of interfamily rivalry: Jaffrey Pyncheon is the present-day embodiment of Colonel Pyncheon. Holgrave exclaims to Phoebe: "[T]he original perpetrator and father of this mischief appears to have perpetuated himself, and still walks the street" (p. 185). Matthew Maule and his dispossessed progeny, including Holgrave, were the victims of this "mischief." There is much more at stake than the Oedipal struggle of a young man against a father figure. Thus, the history of bitter conflict between Pyncheon and Maule, which constitutes the warp and woof of *The House of the Seven Gables*, is being enacted in the present between these two men. Destiny, as it turns out, has arranged that Holgrave, himself, and Jaffrey Pyncheon are the protagonists in this final act of this multigenerational drama. A consideration of Holgrave's personal and family history, which should be the foundation of any psychoanalytic formulation of his crisis, is missing from Crews's interpretation.[2]

Nancy J. Chodorow's (1999) approach serves as a corrective to Crews's exercise of "wild psychoanalysis." She contrasts psychoanalytic epistemology with that of other humanistic disciplines in that it is "first and foremost an account and theory of personal meaning" (p. 129) that employs its technique toward unraveling "the particularistic uniqueness of each individual psyche and life history" (p. 2). In order to comprehend this scene accurately and comprehensively, I will, following Chodorow's lead, contextualize Holgrave's crisis within a psychoanalytically informed, particularistic narrative of his life history, which will ultimately serve as a foundation for interpretations of both the unconscious and the conscious aspects of his transformation. Although Holgrave is but one of the quartet of interesting characters who inhabits the House of the Seven Gables, Hawthorne does provide an abundance of psychological data about him so as to permit the construction of such a narrative. I will conclude that, in the proximity of Jaffrey's dead body, Holgrave confronts both formidable existential anxieties and unconscious conflicts related to a participant role as a Maule in the final chapter of the tormented history of the House of the Seven Gables. In this mutative period of intense contemplation, Holgrave acquires the wisdom of experience but at the cost of a painful loss of youthful innocence for which love with Phoebe, uniquely, can compensate. This wisdom informs the moral, social, and spiritual outlook embraced by the romance's conclusion.

Before proceeding with Holgrave's narrative below, the reader of this chapter will benefit from an explanatory note: this is essentially a cross-discipline study that applies the insights of psychoanalysis to a literary text; therefore, it does not read like an essay written within the genre of literary criticism. As Chodorow avers, the psychoanalytic voice is distinct, and its mode of discourse differs from those that are expressions of other frameworks of literary analysis. The psychoanalytic method generates an argument that builds incrementally from observation to inference and finally to synthetic interpretation. Paul Keegan (2017) is correct in his judgment that "[p]sychoanalysis sets out to show rather than tell, and to redress the immemorial injury of speaking for the subject" (p. 5). In the slow unfolding of Holgrave's "particularistic uniqueness" toward an understanding of his transformation, and in my reliance on extensive quotations from the text in the service of rendering a more objective account of his psychology, I ask of the reader something akin to the narrator's appeal in *The House of the Seven Gables*: "The author needs great faith in his reader's sympathy; else he must hesitate to give details so minute, and incidents apparently so trifling, as are essential to make up the idea of this garden-life" (Vol. 2, 150). Phoebe anticipates our analytic efforts: as Holgrave's relationship with her develops, not unlike that of an analysand to his analyst, during their interchanges in the garden, his chilly reserve is surmounted as he unfolds the story of his life to her. Phoebe possesses those characteristics of "native sagacity," "intuition," "no intrusive egotism," and "sympathy" that, in *The Scarlet Letter* (Hawthorne, 1962, Vol. 1, p. 124), Hawthorne specifies that a physician must possess in order to win the trust of his patient and finally to unlock the secrets of his heart. We will do well in the analysis that follows to emulate Phoebe.

Young Holgrave

Whenever possible, a psychoanalytic inquiry begins with childhood, when, as Freud and generations of psychoanalysts after him have shown, the foundations of enduring psychic structure are formed. This section will generate a psychological portrait of Holgrave before he first crossed the portals of the House of the Seven Gables, which, it is well to remember, was at the tender age of twenty one. Of his past, we are told that "left to his own guidance, he had begun to be self-dependent yet as a boy, and it was aptly suited to his natural force of will" (Vol. 2, p. 176). Thus, it would seem that Holgrave was figuratively or literally orphaned at an early age, always a trauma for any child, whatever may be his natural disposition to autonomy. In having experienced early parental loss, Holgrave joins *The Blithedale Romance*'s half-sisters, Zenobia and Priscilla, and *The Marble Faun*'s Miriam, as well as, of course, Hawthorne himself. Holgrave, without siblings or relatives, is the last surviving Maule and, as such, he has the considerable burden of carrying the full weight of the last link in the Maule family chain. His sole inheritance as a Maule, so he ultimately tells Phoebe, is the knowledge of the location of the hidden Maine land deed, which, intangible legacy that this secret may seem, carries the entire history of the Pyncheons' obsession to acquire the vast property and the Maules' vengeful obstruction of that dream.

As a Maule, whose family fate was to survive on the margin of society, Holgrave was of humble origins, had a scant education, and by his wandering and assumption of a kaleidoscopic variety of occupations, showed no evidence of attachment to place, or, it would seem, to persons. In the lack of solid attachments, one can perhaps discern the influence of early parental loss. With no fixed home, he had been thrown back on inner resources, and in the face of "the many tests which tried his metal," he had developed what can only be characterized as an extraordinarily admirable character (p. 181). Endowed with "efficacy," "personal ambition," "so much faith in himself," "generous impulses," and an "enthusiasm … which gave warmth to everything he laid his hand on," he could eventually bring these strengths in service of his "magnanimous zeal for man's welfare" as a potential "champion of some practicable cause" (pp. 180–181). And, with a trait that has acute relevance, the narrator stresses that, "[h]omeless as he had been—continually changing his whereabout and therefore responsibility to neither public opinion nor to individuals … he never violated the innermost man but carried his conscience along with him" (p. 177). True to his character, Holgrave will ultimately bring this conscience to bear on the moral challenges of his later encounters with both Phoebe and Jaffrey. In all significant ways, Holgrave is an antithesis of his antagonist, Jaffrey, who is exclusively attuned to public opinion and whose lack of conscience puts him in constant violation of his innermost self.

The narrator's listing of Holgrave's geographically scattered employments is whimsical but also telling because, amongst these, we discern several overlaps with Hawthorne's early career. Both the author and Holgrave had been artists in "narrow circumstances" (p. 84) and, having "to earn his bread," (p. 177) had at one time been editors of local publications, as well as writers who published articles and stories in several journals; specifically, both could boast publications in *Godey's Ladies Book and Magazine* and *Graham's Magazine*. In terms of youthful social consciousness, Hawthorne had lived for six months at Brook Farm commune; in a similar spirit, Holgrave "had spent some months in a community of Fourierists" (p. 176). The daguerreotypist's associates, "reformers, temperance-lecturers, and all manner of cross-looking philanthropists" (p. 84), bear a family resemblance to Hawthorne's intellectual coterie in Concord. I think that in these ways, and in others to be mentioned later, Hawthorne identifies with Holgrave more closely than with any other character in his fiction.

After his "conversion," the narrator refers to the daguerreotypist with a friendly sarcasm as "that sworn foe of wealth and all manner of conservatism—the wild reformer—Holgrave!" (p. 313). Holgrave has indeed been passionate in his advocacy of radical social reform. The fate of Holgrave's reformist program and its limitations were forecast by Hawthorne in an earlier work, "The Hall of Fantasy" (1843). In this sketch, the narrator espies a group of reformers who, not unlike Holgrave, "were the representatives of an unquiet period, when mankind is seeking to cast off the whole tissue of ancient custom, like a tattered garment;" he then levels his critique at the narrowness of their vision: "Many of them had gotten possession of some crystal fragment of truth, the brightness of which so dazzled them, that they could see nothing else in the wide universe" (Vol. 10, 180). So the narrator of *The House of the Seven Gables*, although in sympathy with Holgrave's aspiration "as to the better centuries that are coming," employs the same metaphor for the past and stresses that Holgrave's "error lay, in supposing that this age, more than any past or future one, is destined to see the tattered garments of Antiquity exchanged for a new suit, instead of gradually renewing themselves by patchwork" (p. 180). Because of the nature of the human heart, social change, the narrator cautions, can be only evolutionary—not revolutionary. In the "Hall of Fantasy," the narrator professes that "what is good and true becomes gradually hardened into fact, while error melts away and vanishes among the shadows of the hall" (Vol. 10, p. 180). So, too, the narrator of *The House of the Seven Gables* predicts that, with maturity, there will be a gradual evolution in Holgrave's radical views: "And when, with the years settling down more weightily upon him, his earlier faith should be modified by inevitable experience, it would be with no harsh and sudden revolution in his sentiments" (Vol. I0, p. 180). As it turns out, the temporal constraints of the romance do not allow Holgrave the years to do their office in modifying his beliefs; in his confrontation with Jaffrey Pyncheon's corpse, the experience of years is markedly condensed and settles suddenly upon him, and with almost crushing weight.

Holgrave's impulse to reform the present is a measure of his aversion to the past, of which the House of the Seven Gables represents an exemplar. Phoebe is sensitive to this aspect of Holgrave's psychology: "How you hate everything old!" (Vol. 2, p. 184). The artist opines that the "Past ... lies upon the Present like a giant's dead body!" (p. 182). Holgrave, it would seem, shares Hawthorne's proclivity for allegory in casting "that odious and abominable Past" in the image of a "Dead Man" whom he urgently wants to throw off (pp. 183–184): "Shall we never, never get rid of this Past!" (p. 182). The wish is peremptory but will prove unattainable; Holgrave unknowingly foresees what will come to pass in his fearful encounter with Jaffrey: "Turn our eyes to what point we may, a Dead Man's white, immitigable face encounters them, and freezes our very heart!" (p. 183).

Holgrave's railings against the abuses of property were heard earlier in "Earth's Holocaust" (1844): "There was then a cry, that the period was arrived, when the title-deeds of landed property should be given to the flames, and the whole soil of the earth revert to the public, from which it has been wrongfully abstracted, and most unequally distributed among individuals" (Vol. 10, 394). Holgrave comes honestly, and with youthful conviction, by his socialist views. His forefather had been condemned to death, and his family's plot of land had been "wrongfully abstracted" in service of the Pyncheon's powerful will to "plant a family," which he concludes has resulted in the calamity through "a portion of three centuries ... of perpetual remorse of conscience, a constantly defeated hope, strife amongst kindred, various misery ... unspeakable disgrace ..." (Vol. 2, p. 185). Holgrave knows every detail of the Pyncheon/Maule strife, which the narrator relates in the opening chapter of the novel. His passionate disavowal of property rights is not the product of mere intellectual musing but is grounded in painful family history. This passion, however understandable, is narrowly founded on his family's unfortunate experience and results in the vehement quality of his categorical assertion to Phoebe against the idea of building a house for posterity: "I speak true thoughts to a true mind! ... The truth is as I say!" (p. 185). Hawthorne, a perennial foe of doctrine that cloaks itself as truth, will not let this avowal stand unchallenged. Holgrave's youthful dogmatism will be modulated when, in light of his loving relationship with Phoebe and in consideration of their prospective future, he finds sufficient reason to endorse the concept of planting a family of his own.

Holgrave at the House of the Seven Gables

Holgrave brings considerable strengths and vulnerabilities with him to the House of the Seven Gables. This section details the psychological themes revealed by his developing relationships with its inhabitants—Hepzibah, Clifford, and Phoebe—and serves as a prelude to the portentous encounter with Jaffrey Pyncheon's corpse during which the hitherto-tightly-woven strands of his psychology acutely unravel.

Undoubtedly Holgrave had arrived at the House of the Seven Gables and appealed to Hepzibah as a young artist looking for a room to rent; if she had known he was a Maule, there would have been "no vacancy." She well knew the malice that the Maules bore toward her family. Holgrave was careful to hide his identity and his resentments: "The Maules, at all events, kept their resentments within their own breasts" (p. 4). Although concealed, they were kept alive and festered. This unresolved resentment and wish for revenge fuels the repetition compulsion that Holgrave enacts in returning to the site of the crime against his family.[3] The Maules had many ways to exact their revenge, including exercising nefarious influence on the Pyncheons: It was said that Old Matthew Maule, "the ghostly creditor, would have his finger in all the affairs of the Pyncheons, and make everything go wrong with them" (p. 189). The Maules were also said to influence the House's looking glass, in which the Pyncheons would appear "as doing over and again some deed of sin, or in the crisis of life's bitterest sorrow" (p. 21). Moreover, the memory of the Pyncheon sin is kept alive since the Maules serve as an externalization of a punitive superego: "Matthew Maule … trode downward from his own age to a far later one, planting a heavy footstep, all the way, on the conscience of a Pyncheon" (p. 20). Thus, there is a great deal more to Holgrave's motivation to live in enemy territory, as it is freighted with personal meaning, as he obliquely expresses in his guarded reply to Phoebe's inquiry as to his purpose in the House: "Oh, I am pursuing my studies here; not in books, however!" (p. 184). Holgrave has come to haunt the House of the Seven Gables; however, he will learn that the legacy of these destructive wishes and their baleful influence have taken up residence in his own haunted mind.

Holgrave with Hepzibah and Clifford

Holgrave has lived for three months in the House of the Seven Gables before Hepzibah opens her penny-shop and he is on cordial terms with her. In fact, she is drawn to him as a person who "has such a way of taking hold of one's mind" (p. 85) and considers him "her only friend" (p. 46). Holgrave makes a point to be her first customer and the first who offers to put money in her hand. Although he states that he is there to "merely look in, to offer my best wishes," (p. 43) there is also a Maule agenda at work in his participation at the very moment of her social debasement "when the patrician lady is to be transformed into the plebian woman" (p. 38). For Hepzibah, this is indeed something of a "crisis of life's bitterest sorrows" and Holgrave, the Maule in attendance, derives sadistically tinged, voyeuristic pleasure from the scene.[4] Hepzibah comments to Holgrave: "But I am a woman … I was going to say a lady,—but I consider that as past" (p. 44). Holgrave answers, "'Well; no matter if it be past!' … *a strange gleam of half-hidden sarcasm flashing through the kindliness of his manner*" (p. 44; emphasis added). And in a stroke of narratorial irony, there is more truth to Hepzibah's subsequent comment than she realizes: "[I]f old Maule's host, or a descendent of his, could see me behind the counter to-day, he would call it the fulfillment of his worst wishes" (p. 46). Holgrave is at the moment gratifying those very wishes.

In order to have access to his uncle's fortune after his sudden death, Jaffrey Pyncheon framed Clifford, whose resulting imprisonment in solitary confinement for three decades, as I have shown elsewhere, resulted in psychic trauma of unimaginable proportions.[5] Clifford returns to the House of the Seven Gables virtually broken, mentally, emotionally, and spiritually. He is a marginally surviving victim of the "pure and uncontrollable mischief" that has turned Pyncheon against Pyncheon in the pursuit of "ill-gotten gold" (p. 2). His presence in the House is a constant reminder of the terrible cost of the destructiveness of human greed. In fact, word for word and paragraph for paragraph, Clifford's disjointed states of mind take up more of the novel's narrative than any other subject. As the object of love and devotion from both Hepzibah and Phoebe and due to their tireless ministrations, he is gradually nurtured into a significant, albeit partial, recovery from his mental disabilities. Hawthorne, I believe, uses the response to Clifford's suffering as the measure of his characters' moral stature. Hepzibah, often the object of the narrator's charitable derision, gets the highest rating: "[S]he had kept her faith, alone of all the world, wholly, unfaulteringly, at every instant, and throughout life. And here, in his late decline, the lost one had come back out of his long and strange misfortune, and was thrown on her sympathy, as it seemed, not merely for the bread of his physical existence, but for everything that should keep him morally alive. She had responded to the call!" (p. 133). Phoebe becomes Hepzibah's deputy in the rehabilitative effort since her youthful manner and unfailing instincts are so salutary to the broken man: "[S]he discerned what was good for him, and did it" (p. 143). She performs exemplary service with great sensitivity and empathy for his plight, which she expresses to the artist: "He has had such a great sorrow, that his heart is made all solemn and sacred by it" (p. 178).

Not so for Holgrave. Clifford is an object of great interest to him, but he is not the recipient of his empathy. Regarding the Malbone portrait of a young Clifford, he comments: "It will suit my purpose still better, to see the original" (p. 93). And when he did interact with Clifford, he "took some pains to establish an intercourse" with him (p. 156); but the narrator betrays Holgrave's Maule agenda, which holds Clifford as an object of voyeuristic curiosity: "In the artist's deep, thoughtful, all-observant eyes, there was now-and-then an expression, not sinister, but questionable; as if he had some other interest in the scene than a stranger, a youthful and unconnected adventurer might be supposed to have" (p. 156). Phoebe is aware of Holgrave's detachment: "Phoebe felt his eye, often; his heart, seldom or never. He took a certain kind interest in Hepzibah and her brother … but, after all, he never exactly made common cause with them, nor gave any reliable evidence that he loved them better, in proportion as he knew them more … he cared nothing for them, or comparatively so little, as objects of human affection" (pp. 177–178). Holgrave, it would seem, is moved to participate in the "united struggle of mankind" (p. 45), but cannot join in common cause with the victims of misfortune, Pyncheons though they might be. In the face of such suffering, Holgrave's curiosity has an almost cruel quality. For Phoebe, Clifford's sorrow constitutes "holy ground where the shadow falls!" (p. 178), a respect for which restrains her from penetrating any further. Holgrave has no such inhibition: "Had I your opportunities, no scruples would prevent me from fathoming Clifford to the full depth of my plummet-line!" (p. 178). Maule resentment obstructs empathy toward a most unfortunate and innocent Pyncheon. Here Holgrave, in his aggressive insensitivity, is contemplating one of the gravest in Hawthorne's hierarchy of human crimes, the violation of the human heart. This insensitivity will soon bring about a rift between him and Phoebe.

Holgrave and Phoebe

In his reserve, and his eschewing of intimacy, Holgrave shares the psychological legacy of the Maules whose "companions, or those who endeavored to become such, grew conscious of a circle roundabout [them] … within the sanctity or spell of which … it was impossible for any man to step" (p. 26). Employing architecture as a metaphor for the psyche, the narrator tells that Holgrave took up residence "in a remote gable—quite a house by itself, indeed—with locks, bolts and oaken bars on all intervening doors" (p. 30). Phoebe senses these restraints: "[S]he scarcely thought him affectionate in nature. He was too calm and cool an observer. Phoebe felt his eye, often; his heart, seldom or never" (p. 177). Thus, the daguerreotypist's deepening relationship with Phoebe, in which his formidable emotional barriers are surmounted, must be considered a spectacular psychological achievement, and, of course, a tribute to Phoebe's "kind of natural magic … to bring out the hidden capabilities of things" (p. 71).

Initially, Holgrave is wary about Phoebe, and at their first encounter, he evokes the familiar battle lines between Maule and Pyncheon: "For you are a Pyncheon?" (p. 90). They gradually become acquainted and their joint cultivation of the garden is a sign of an ultimate compatibility. However, Holgrave misreads Phoebe: "With the insight on which he prided himself, he fancied he could look through Phoebe, and all around her, and could read her off like the pages of a child's story-book" (p. 182). To the contrary, the narrator instructs us: "But these transparent natures are often deceptive with their depth" (p. 182). So it is with Phoebe, whose profound humanity and loving generosity bring joy, comfort, and healing to all those around her. With no questions asked, she comes to Hepzibah's assistance with alacrity; her sensitivity and infallible instincts enable her to provide Clifford with just the right kind of stimulation that promotes the reintegration of the fragments of his disordered psyche. Uncle Venner, Ned Higgins, the wandering Italian barrel-organ player, and even the backyard chickens who alight on her shoulder are all magnetically drawn in by her homely witchcraft.

Holgrave falls victim to Phoebe's natural sympathy and all that goes with it. Hitherto homeless, shiftless, and apparently without intimate relationships, he becomes deeply attached to Phoebe: "Without such purpose, on her part, and unconsciously on his, she made the House of the Seven Gables like a home to him, and the garden a familiar precinct" (p. 182).[6] Phoebe's ability as a listener would be the envy of any psychoanalyst: "Thus the artist, whatever he might judge of Phoebe's capacity, was beguiled, by some silent charm of hers, to talk freely of what he dreamed of doing in the world. He poured himself out as to another self ... and was moved only by the inevitable tendency of thought, when rendered sympathetic by enthusiasm and emotion, to flow to the first safe reservoir it finds" (p. 182). For her to make the hated House of the Seven Gables into a home for him bespeaks her transformative charm, which has the quality of a "spiritual force" (p. 137). The narrator invites us to participate, as voyeurs, in a vignette that betrays Holgrave's hidden affection: "But, had you peeped at them through the chinks in the garden-fence, the young man's earnestness and heightened color might have led you to suppose that he was making love to the young girl!" (p. 182).

The Legend of Alice Pyncheon

Holgrave comes to the House of the Seven Gables to witness Pyncheon destruction, and seer though he may be, he does not reckon that within its confines he will fall in love with a Pyncheon woman. Since he "habitually masked whatever lay near his heart" (p. 301), we can suspect that he is not aware of the depths of his feelings for Phoebe; that will come later. However, in matters of passion, one cannot deceive the unconscious. Love and hate toward the Pyncheons have taken up uneasy co-residence in Holgrave's psyche and produced significant unconscious conflict that is manifest symptomatically as obsession: "I believe I am a little mad!" he admits to Phoebe: "This subject has taken hold of my mind with the strangest tenacity of clutch, since I have lodged in yonder old gable. As one method of throwing it off, I have put an incident in the Pyncheon family-history, with which I happen to be acquainted, into the form of a legend, and mean to publish it in a magazine" (p. 186). Through writing, Holgrave is attempting to sublimate intrapsychic conflict; this serves as a fertile clue as to the dynamics of Hawthorne's creativity.

In having penned the legend of Alice Pyncheon, Holgrave, at a crossroads, takes center stage in the romance. Although there are hints of the sad story of Alice Pyncheon that Hepzibah has retold to Phoebe with regard to the family harpsichord, the legend is essentially Holgrave's creation, and it is pure Hawthornian tale-writing. Hawthorne may distance himself from Holgrave by stressing that he is a visual artist, a daguerreotypist, of uncertain promise, but as the tale demonstrates, Holgrave, "who appeared to have a literary turn," is also an accomplished writer (p. 145). Thus, the identification that Hawthorne, having achieved fame as the author of *The Scarlet Letter*, has with young Holgrave helps account for the extraordinary care with which this character is rendered. The legend, like a dream in which the unconscious can be decoded, reveals what is stirred up in Holgrave's psyche as he is drawn into an intense relationship with Phoebe. It is a cautionary tale of the danger of sexual attraction that risks rejection and retaliation. Through the legend, sexuality is injected, for the first time, into the long history of the Maule/Pyncheon brew of greed and revenge.

Like Matthew Maule's being called to the House of the Seven Gables and entering a complex relationship with Alice, so Holgrave is drawn there and is involved with Phoebe. Matthew Maule is obviously smitten with Alice and feels degraded by her reacting to his physical attractiveness but to nothing more. Alice is a patrician who is "set apart from the world's vulgar mass" (p. 201), and Maule is, after all, a plebian. The resentment that Maule feels at the wide class distinction echoes the history of exploitation by the socially powerful Pyncheons over the lowly Maules; Holgrave also comes to the House with a chip on his shoulder as to the social privilege of the wealthy, and as we have seen, this disparity conditioned the radical nature of his social philosophy.[7] Maule's resentment rises to rage when he experiences what he interprets as humiliation by Alice. Although Alice's "pride" is at issue, and something she pays for with her life, Matthew Maule's vulnerability to narcissistic injury is the more prominent feature of the tale. The horrific outcome of the story is determined when, in one solitary glance by Alice, Matthew Maule, with exquisitely poised sensitivity, reads his rejection in the young woman's condescension:

> [H]er eyes fell upon the carpenter … clad in … a pair of loose breeches open at the knees, and with a long pocket for his rule, the end of which protruded; it was a proper mark of his artizan calling.… A glow of artistic approval brightened over Alice Pyncheon's face … of the remarkable comeliness, strength and energy of Maule's figure. But that admiring glance … the carpenter never forgave … the devil himself made Maule so subtile in his perception (p. 201).[8]

As in the scene at the precipice of the Tarpeian Rock in *The Marble Faun*, the entire tragedy is propelled by the reading of one unguarded glance. Alice's "pride" is undoubtedly in large part the product of her privileged upbringing and superior European education but is mitigated by her innate tenderness: "For the sake of that redeeming quality, a man of generous nature would have almost forgiven all her pride, and been content, almost, to lie down in her path, and let Alice set her slender foot upon his heart. All that he would have required was simply the acknowledgement that he was indeed a man, and a fellow-being, moulded of the same elements as she" (p. 201). This is not the case. Matthew Maule does not have a generous nature, and he reacts to Alice's aloofness as if she did not consider him of her same substance. The perceived personal slight, reinforced by the history of the ill-treatment of the

Maules by the Pyncheons, ignites Matthew Maule's overwhelming wish for revenge. Much could be written about the mesmeric interchange between Maule, Alice, and her father. Suffice it to say that Alice, in her innocence, does not adequately reckon on the strength of unconscious forces in the mental contest in which she submits herself to Maule, or on the greed that occasions her father to abandon her, if only for a few seconds, to Maule's control. She falls victim to Maule's domination, in which she is sadistically subjected to repeated and, finally, to fatal, degradation. Matthew Maule's actions against Alice constitute another instance of the "pure and uncontrollable mischief" plaguing the interfamily conflict (p. 2). Although a Maule himself, Holgrave, the author of the tale, herein concedes that abundant evil can flow from the Maule side of the conflict. Neither does Matthew Maule gain anything other than the indulgence of sadistic pleasure in his domination of Alice nor is it made clear that he has remorse at her death: "He is the darkest and wofullest man that ever walked behind a corpse. He had meant to humble Alice, not to kill her" (p. 210).[9] Not unlike the case of Dimmesdale's victimization by Chillingworth in *The Scarlet Letter*, only death releases Alice from Maule's fiendish thrall.

The story of Alice Pyncheon is a tragic one, since it involves the degradation and death of an essentially moral and innocent woman, albeit one whose *hamartia* was maiden pride. However, the punishment does not fit the crime: the legend of Alice Pyncheon is arguably the most gratuitously cruel in all Hawthorne's oeuvre, and he cannily channels this tale through Holgrave's pen. One does not need to be a psychoanalyst to propose that Holgrave's unconscious desire to dominate a woman is folded into the sadism of his character, Matthew Maule. His growing erotic tie to Phoebe has aroused the desire to take pleasure in subjugation and control, as the narrator somewhat abstractly comments: "[T]here is no temptation so great as the opportunity of acquiring empire over the human spirit; nor any idea more seductive to a young man, than to become the arbiter of a young girl's destiny" (p. 212). Alice dies after she is called to attend to Maule's bride at their wedding; the tale teaches that a man cannot have a loving bride and possess a woman-slave. Through this legend, Holgrave is expressing the psychological conundrum aroused by his deepening relationship to Phoebe: he cannot both possess and love her; it is one or the other.[10]

Holgrave is immediately put to the test as Phoebe is mesmerized by his recitation of the legend. The confrontation between Matthew Maule and Alice Pyncheon is brought alive into the present moment between Holgrave and Phoebe. Like Alice, Phoebe has submitted herself to a Maule's magnetic influence. Here, Holgrave's strength of character and respect for the individuality of the other overcomes his dark desires. That he "forbade himself to twine that one link more, which might have rendered his spell over Phoebe indissoluble" (p. 212), indicates both the mental conflict and a conscious moral decision not to take possession of her.[11] The integrity of Holgrave's conscience, for which he has already received the narrator's praise, overcomes the compulsion to replicate Matthew Maule's crime against Alice Pyncheon. In this way, Holgrave frees himself from the weight of the past. Freud's repetition compulsion has been overcome so that release and regeneration may be possible. This decision constitutes the first but decisive step in the dissolution of the curse of the House of the Seven Gables.

In successfully passing this test of character, a *rite de passage*, Holgrave has been readied to enter the portal of enchantment brought about by romance. In the garden he and Phoebe linger to observe that "the sun had gone down and was tinting the clouds toward the zenith with those bright hues which are not seen until some time after sunset" (pp. 212–213). The light of the rising moon was "already powerful enough to change the character of the lingering daylight … the artist chanced to be one, on whom the reviving influence fell. It made him feel—what he sometimes almost forgot, thrust early, as he had been, into the rude struggle of man with man—how young he still was" (p. 213). Holgrave muses: "Could I keep the feeling that now possesses me, the garden would every day be virgin soil … and the house!—it would be like a bower in Eden, blossoming with the earliest roses that God ever made" (p. 214). Holgrave's associations to his feelings betray that he, like a new Adam, is under the spell of his Eve, Phoebe. Holgrave and the narrator think alike: the imagery of the Garden of Eden is identical to the imagery that the narrator will employ in describing his union with Phoebe after his crisis. Holgrave is not aware that Phoebe is the source of the romantic bliss that he feels, but he accurately assesses that this unique realm of feeling has the power to transform his drive as a radical reformer: "Moonlight, and the sentiment in men's heart, responsive to it, is the greatest of renovators and reformers. All other reform and renovation, I suppose, will prove no better than moonshine!" (p. 214). Contrary to Von Abele's (1955) contention that Holgrave's "conversion" from radical to conservative "is scarcely prepared for in the book" (p. 59), its psychological foundation is set in this passage.

Holgrave has to surmount a further trial, however, before he will merit an enduring happiness with Phoebe; as in a fairy tale, of which, as Dennis R. Perry (2014) points out, there are many elements in *The House of the Seven Gables,* the hero must do battle to the death with an adversary before he can rightly claim the heroine. Although Holgrave has neutralized the destructive instincts that might threaten the womanhood of Phoebe, he needs to reform the Maule malevolence that he still holds toward others in the Pyncheon family. It is Phoebe who tells him so in no uncertain terms. In relation to her imminent departure from the House, Holgrave predicts a dire influence on her elderly cousins: as for Clifford, "I should not wonder if he were to crumble away," and Hepzibah "will lose what little flexibility she has" (p. 216). He speaks unflatteringly, saying that Hepzibah "is in fact dead; although she galvanizes herself into a semblance of life, and stands behind her counter, afflicting the world with a greatly-to-be-deprecated scowl" (216). He refers to "the imbecile, branded, half-torpid Clifford" (p. 218) as "another dead and long-buried person … this degraded and shattered gentleman—this abortive lover of the Beautiful" (p. 216). Phoebe, who is committed to her cousins' welfare, reacts pointedly to these derogatory descriptions: "Mr. Holgrave, I am sometimes puzzled to know whether you wish them well or ill" (p. 216). Thus, Phoebe's comment ushers in an interchange with Holgrave that breaks their spell of enchantment.

In telling Phoebe of his premonition of the oncoming crisis between Clifford and Jaffrey, Holgrave again reveals to her an unseemly sort of voyeurism: "It is not my impulse—as regarding these two individuals—either to help or hinder; but to look on, to analyze, to explain matters to myself, and to comprehend the drama which, for almost two hundred years has been dragging its slow length over the ground.... If permitted to witness the close, I doubt not to derive moral satisfaction from it, go matters how they may" (pp. 216–217). Phoebe is quick to appreciate the heartlessness of Holgrave's position and her remonstrance is devastating:

> I wish you would speak more plainly ... and, above all, that you would feel more like a christian and a human being! How is it possible to see people in distress, without desiring, more than anything else, to help and comfort them? You talk as if this old house were a theatre: and you seem to look at Hepzibah and Clifford's misfortunes, and those of generations before them, as a tragedy, such as I have seen acted in the hall of a country-hotel; only the present one appears to be played exclusively for your amusement. I do not like this. The play costs the performers too much—and the audience is too cold-hearted! (p. 217)

Lest there be any doubt, Phoebe is not all sweetness and light; her pungent retort enforces a clearheaded moral authority. Clifford is a pathetic victim of long injustice, and Jaffrey is the powerful and unrepentant perpetrator. In such a situation, there is no question as to where moral sentiments and sympathies must lie; Holgrave's condescending neutrality just will not do. Whatever past resentment he holds toward the Pyncheon family needs to be overcome if he is to respond to this severely imbalanced confrontation with a requisite empathy and succor, and, I would suggest, to be worthy to regain Phoebe's loving regard. Her exhortation that Holgrave "feel more like a christian and a human being" is an unsparing critique of a moral failing. She is angry with him and there is a rift which he senses: "'Then let us part friends!' said Holgrave pressing her hand. 'Or if not as friends, let us part before you entirely hate me. You, who love everybody else in the world!'" (p. 218). In the face of this falling out with Phoebe and his separation from her brought about by her imminent departure from the House of the Seven Gables, Holgrave has much to ponder. In the realm of emotions, Holgrave is cut off from "the first safe reservoir" that he ever found (p. 182). What he states to Phoebe as true of Hepzibah and Clifford is equally true of himself: "Whatever health, comfort, and natural life, exists in this house, is embodied in your person.... They both exist by you!" (p. 216). Holgrave's striking reaction to Phoebe's reappearance in the House must be understood in light of the dependence on her that he has already developed and the breach that he has recently experienced. Immediately after Phoebe's departure, a severe easterly storm settles in, and the narrator's comment on the House's hearth can equally be interpreted as descriptive of the condition of Holgrave's heart, bereft of Phoebe: "[T]he great kitchen-fireplace, which served all the better as an emblem of the mansion's heart … though built for warmth … was now so comfortless and empty" (p. 224).

Crisis: Holgrave and Governor Pyncheon

Our narrative about Holgrave is reaching the decisive scene; however, two confrontations with Jaffrey Pyncheon's corpse precede his. The first is Clifford's, whose manic reaction of release from his nemesis propels him, and Hepzibah with him, out of the House and on a railway journey to nowhere. The second is the narrator's in the peerless Chapter XVIII, "Governor Pyncheon." I will suggest that this chapter's tonal movement from mockery to terror to hope serves as a template for Holgrave's psychological journey in the presence of the body the next morning. In "Governor Pyncheon," the narrator approaches the Judge as one who, coming into the parlor and spying his sedentary body, addresses him as if he were still alive: "Make haste, then! Do your part! The meed for which you have toiled, and fought, and climbed, and crept, is ready for your grasp!" (p. 274). This conceit is sustained through the scene and serves as the ironic foundation for savage mockery and hostility. Essentially, by pretending that Jaffrey is still alive, the narrator is playing with the dead, and in addressing the reader in the collective "we," the narrator offers an invitation to participate in the desecration. The unsurpassed brilliance of the satiric mode allows us to forget, for the moment, that we are irreverently gloating over a corpse. If we are true to ourselves, we may admit that we read this scene with genuine, albeit guilty, pleasure. Gathered around Jaffrey's dead body, we are enlisted as avenging, demonic Maule spirits. Our own sadism is engaged in a scene that brings us into the forbidden region of necrophilia.

As time passes, however, the ghoulishly humorous mode yields to a tone of increasing angst. As Jaffrey's visage is effaced by the failing daylight, its specificity as belonging to one uniquely cruel man, morphs into the abstracted face of immutable Death.

No longer disembodied voyeurs, we become participants in the existential terror of the scene: "An infinite, inscrutable blackness has annihilated sight! Where is our universe? All crumbling away from ours; and we, adrift in chaos, may harken to the gusts of homeless winds, that go sighing and murmuring about us, in quest of what was once a world!" (pp. 276–277). In all this confused sensory experience, we are cut loose from familiar moorings and become disoriented. The sound of Jaffrey's watch, signaling the pace of the inexorable march to death, crowns the scene: "Be the cause what it may, this little, quiet, never-ceasing throb of Time's pulse, repeating its small strokes with such busy regularity, in Judge Pyncheon's motionless hand, has an effect of terror, which we do not find in any other accompaniment of the scene" (p. 277). Now victims of our own reckless indulgence, we have been led into an unanticipated face-off with the great enemies, in allegorical form, of our mortal condition, Time and Death. No longer wishing to linger in what has been sport, we are in haste to flee: "Would that we were not an attendant spirit, here! It is too awful!" (pp. 277–278). The Judge's inert body and the confrontations that it has foisted upon us bring us to the point of psychological breakdown: "Will he never stir again? We shall go mad, unless he stirs!" (p. 281).

Although Jaffrey Pyncheon is dead, with the daylight, the living world awakens around his lifeless form. As R. A. Yoder (1974) points out, "[T]he importance of time passing, of the evolutionary movement that governs the book, is established symbolically by means of the diurnal cycle" (p. 46). The terror of the night just past yields to dawn and a rebirth of hope: "But the great world-clock of Time still keeps its beat. The dreary night—for, Oh, how dreary seems its haunted waste, behind us!—gives place to a fresh, transparent, cloudless morn. Blessed, blessed, radiance! The day-beam … seems part of the universal benediction, annulling evil, and rendering all goodness possible, and happiness attainable" (pp. 281–282). The profane Walpurgisnacht transmutes into an allegory of sunrise with the spiritual possibilities of renewal and redemption. This is an important instance of what John Gatta Jr. (1978) perceptively characterizes as the romance's "transhistorical, figurative level of narrative recognizable in traditional Christian terms as sacred or visionary history" (p. 38).

A few hours after dawn, Holgrave's encounter with Jaffrey's corpse will follow a similar ascending arc from darkness to radiant light. As a way to indicate its significance, the text is specific about when Holgrave finds Jaffrey: the inner door to the parlor, closed when Ned Higgins tries to gain access to the House, is open when the butcher peers in through a little window in the outer door. In the interval between these two morning visitors, Holgrave has entered the parlor. He recounts to Phoebe the compulsion that drew him into the chamber: "A feeling which I cannot describe—an indefinite sense of some catastrophe, or consummation—impelled me to make my way into this part of the house, where I discovered what you see" (p. 303).

Holgrave remains with Jaffrey's corpse for an hour. Key elements of the narrator's vigil, which encompasses almost a day, are compressed into this hour. We can imagine that, like the narrator's first view into the parlor, when Holgrave actually crosses the threshold, he is, for a brief while, perplexed as to the Judge's seated pose, especially since the arm is frozen in a lifelike extended position with a watch in his hand. Undoubtedly, with his all-observant eyes, Holgrave soon realizes that Jaffrey is dead. The Judge's "black and damnable" crime against his first cousin, Clifford, was "so great a sin" that a sudden death, at the moment of his ascent to highest state political power, is a fitting destiny (p. 312). Thus, at the most immediate level, the "scene of sin and of retribution worse than guilt," which Holgrave reports to Phoebe, belongs to Jaffrey (p. 306). With the store of hostility that Holgrave holds personally toward the Judge, who is the exemplification of abusive Pyncheon power, it is altogether possible that there is here exaltation and equally savage mockery over the body. Holgrave is capable of this. His viewing of Jaffrey's blood-stained body in the parlor reenacts the visionary scene in his legend of Alice Pyncheon in which "meanly dressed figures," two Maules, "mocked and jeered at the much-abashed old [Pyncheon] dignitary, and pointed their fingers at the stain!" (p. 207). And there is no small amount of sadism expressed in Holgrave's rendering of Gervayse Pyncheon's realization that Alice has been enslaved by Matthew Maule: "Then, it was a strange sight to behold, how the man of conventionalities shook the powder out of his periwig; how the reserved and stately gentleman forgot his dignity; how the gold-embroidered waistcoat flickered and glistened in the firelight, with the convulsion of rage, terror, and sorrow, in the human heart that was beating under it!" (pp. 205–206). The cruelty of this description of a father's grief over his daughter is breathtaking and rivals, as a macabre tour de force, the narrator's rendering of the night vigil.

The phase of mockery is a matter of conjecture, for it is not a part of what Holgrave tells Phoebe. If we allow this surmise, it is possible to imagine that, just as in the narrator's night vigil, the sardonic mood yields to the more ominous and destabilizing aspects of Jaffrey's dead body. It is these that challenge Holgrave to the core and are the starting point of his account to Phoebe of the "dark, cold, miserable hour" before her arrival (p. 306).

In describing it, Holgrave has already expanded the meaning of the scene from what is particular and personal to what is abstract and general: the corpse is referred to as "yonder dead man," not Jaffrey Pyncheon by name; his presence threw a "great black shadow over *everything*" and made "*the universe*, so far as my perceptions could reach, a scene of guilt and of retribution more dreadful than guilt" (p. 306; emphases added). Holgrave has begun to allegorize his experience, and its enlarged meanings are the product of an hour-long, intense contemplation that brings him to conclude: "The sense of it took away my youth. I never hoped to feel young again!" (p. 306).[12] In his report to Phoebe, Holgrave does not narrate the distance he traveled between his perception of Jaffrey's guilt and retribution and the resulting feeling of lost youth. Hawthorne, not uncharacteristically, leaves the responsibility to "fill in the blank" to the empathic imagination of the reader.[13] The reader's participation in this creative work is crucial because the crux of Holgrave's psychological transformation, as I hope to show, is to be found in what has transpired psychologically in this unnamed narrative gap.[14]

Holgrave is a diligent historian of the Pyncheons and Maules; there is nothing the narrator recounts throughout the novel of their troubled histories that Holgrave himself would not have been capable of writing. In essence, the entire weight of the history of the House of the Seven Gables is being brought into his contemplation of Jaffrey's corpse. This is the culmination of the romance, for as the narrator states in the Preface, "The point of view in which this Tale comes under the Romantic definition, lies in the attempt to connect a by-gone time with the very Present that is flitting away from us" (p. 2). No longer enjoying the privilege of a sardonic onlooker, Holgrave is forced by his very presence to participate in the conclusion of the drama. He is the Maule presiding at the last fulfillment of the curse on the Pyncheons: "God will give him blood to drink!" (p. 8). There is the Judge's inert body, and there is the bloodstain on his shirt collar. However, even in the face of the fulfillment of the Maule curse, the contest is not yet over: Jaffrey Pyncheon in death has a power over him that Holgrave did not reckon.

The bygone time has indeed come alive in his mind, and with a vengeance, as it brings with it all its destructive legacies from both the Maule side and the Pyncheon side of the divide: false accusation, persecution, execution, torture, alienation, suspicion, shame, cruel domination, and untimely death. A profusion of images and deep feelings associated with this turbulent history in which he is now an active part, I suggest, overpowers Holgrave's orderly consciousness and colors his imagination. Viewed through this dark historical lens, everything before him is a scene in a larger canvas of guilt and terrible retribution. Similar to the experience of the narrator in "The Haunted Mind," in the proximity of death, "those dark receptacles are flung wide open," and the "buried ones and prisoners" emerge with overwhelming force (Vol. 9, p. 306). The narrator of the sketch is beset with visual, quasi-allegorical fiends that represent past scenes of guilty betrayal, sexual sin, and murder. We are not told of the particular form of the demons that arose from Holgrave's unconscious to be confronted, but what the narrator of "The Haunted Mind" confesses is surely true for the daguerreotypist: "Sufficient without such guilt, is the nightmare of the soul; this heavy, heavy sinking of the spirits, this wintry gloom about the heart; this indistinct horror of the mind, blending with the darkness of the chamber" (Vol. 9, p. 306). Holgrave has peered at the dual fiends of Eros and Thanatos that dwell within, and his bright innocence has been stained by the lurid hue of this experience.

Moreover, as with the band of avenging spirits in the narrator's night vigil, so the presence of "immitigable" Death incites in Holgrave an existential terror. Holgrave's passionate and single-minded attempts to free himself from the past, virtually a modus vivendi, cannot be realized. The weight of the past is inescapably upon him and must always be reckoned with. This brings to mind his earlier lament to Phoebe: "Shall we never get rid of this Past! … It lies upon the present like a giant's dead body! … Turn our eyes to what point we may, a Dead Man's white, immitigable face encounters them, and freezes our very heart!" (pp. 182–183). And, so it does. The omnipresence of the past and its influence on the present also have implications for Holgrave's advocacy of radical social reform. He exclaims to Phoebe in the garden: "Just think, a moment; and it will startle you to see what slaves we are to by-gone times—to

Death, if we give the matter the right word!" (p. 183). Baym's (1970) comment on this passage is insightful:

> The rigid immobility of the corpse turns Holgrave's words back against him, demonstrating that we are indeed slaves to Death. The real existence of death is precisely what foredooms all radical attempts to transfigure reality, and gives the conservative position whatever validity it may have. The judge has escaped his avenger by becoming, finally, Death itself (pp. 596–97).

This confrontation with death, with its converging disruptive emotional reverberations of the past and of immediate existential dislocations, precipitates the loss of Holgrave's first youth.[15] At several points, the narrator stresses Holgrave's youthfulness: he had been "so little harmed, too, by the many tests that had tried his metal," and even "in his premature experience,"(p. 181) he still possessed the "beautiful spirit of youth.... Man's own youth is the world's youth; at least, he feels as if it were, and imagines that the earth's granite substance is something not yet hardened, and which he can mould into whatever shapes he likes. So it was with Holgrave" (p. 179). In his optimism, Holgrave believes that he can ensure that, in his time, the "moss-grown and rotten Past is to be torn down, and lifeless institutions to be thrust out of the way, and their dead corpses buried, and everything to begin anew" (p. 179). His vigil with Jaffrey Pyncheon breaks down that belief. The past and all that goes with it cannot be thrust away but must be lived with. And the earth's granite substance, so he comes to realize, will stubbornly resist efforts to be molded. Therefore, his future, which he believed that he could shape in accordance with his will, becomes, in these moments of realization, "a shapeless gloom, which I must mould into gloomy shapes!" (p. 306). Through her immersion in the suffering of her cousins, Phoebe has already experienced the loss of her youth, more gradually and gracefully, but undeniably, as she reports: "I have grown a great deal older, in this little time. Older, and, I hope, wiser, and—not exactly sadder—but, certainly, with not half so much lightness in my spirits!" (p. 214). Holgrave's loss of youthful innocence, at the hands of "inevitable experience" is more traumatic than Phoebe's (p.180). It proves to involve a "harsh and sudden revolution of his sentiments," which defines the quintessence of his transformation (p. 180).

A loss of the sense of being young brings in its wake a pervasive sense of depression that dominates Holgrave's report to Phoebe. He is no longer protected by the omnipotent fantasies of youth but is thrust out into an oppositional world that, at the time, looks "strange, wild, evil, hostile" (p. 306). The loss must bring with it resonances of other losses that he had suffered. Holgrave has had to survive on his own, as he had been "left to his own guidance" at an early age (p. 176). Whatever losses rendered him so solitary in life had been defended against and compensated for by a sturdy self-reliance. With his confidence shaken and his self-possession loosened, Holgrave must,

I propose, relive painful feelings of being alone, unprotected, and helpless. The emotions related to the breach with Phoebe, a maternal figure, to be sure, reinforces a sense of abandonment. His vulnerability is apparent in his plea to Phoebe: "You must be both strong and wise; for I am all astray, and need your counsel" (pp. 301–302). Acute feelings of depression flood Holgrave and bring him near the point of psychological decompensation.

We have now bridged, psychologically, the narrative gap between Holgrave's perception of a scene of guilt and retribution and his depressed and alienated state. The psychic torments of the narrator in "The Haunted Mind" are assuaged by a fantasy of a loving woman as a companion in his bed: "By desperate effort, you start upright, breaking from a sort of conscious sleep, and gazing wildly round the bed, as if the fiends were anywhere but in your haunted mind.... As your head falls back on the pillow, you think—in a whisper be it spoken—how pleasant in these night solitudes would be the rise and fall of a softer breathing than you own, the slight pressure of a tenderer bosom, the quiet throb of a purer heart, imparting its peacefulness to your troubled one, as if the fond sleeper were involving you in her dream" (Vol. 9, p. 306). Hawthorne is utterly consistent over the intervening years as to the transformative power of a woman's love. As Phoebe crosses the threshold of the House and with Holgrave's grasp of her hand, the fantasy created in "The Haunted Mind" is brought to life, and with it, a smile onto Holgrave's hitherto-troubled face: "It was the look wherewith a man, brooding alone over some fearful object, in a dreary forest, or illimitable desert, would recognize the familiar aspect of his dearest friend, bringing up all the peaceful ideas that belong to home, and the gentle current of every-day affairs" (p. 301). His reunion with Phoebe brings Holgrave home again, with security, comfort, and love. What Hepzibah says to Clifford upon his return to the House is also germane to the daguerreotypist: "There is nothing but love here, Clifford ... nothing but love! You are home!" (pp. 106–107).

Phoebe, bright and shining, as the derivation of her name from the Greek suggests, is the living embodiment of the sunrise after the narrator's night vigil, for she, too, brings with her renewal and redemption. She has transformed the House of the Seven Gables from a place of disease to one of recovery. Through her generous character, she has gone as far as is humanly possible to assist Clifford in recovering from prolonged mental trauma. Although "God is the sole worker of realities," (p. 180) his agent in the House has been Phoebe, who, in Hepzibah's informed estimation, is "one of God's angels" (p. 182). For the daguerreotypist, it is she who renders "all goodness possible, and happiness attainable" (p. 282). In the garden, Holgrave identifies the moonlight as the source of enchantment: "It seems to me ... that I never watched the coming of so beautiful an eve, and never felt anything like happiness as at this moment. After all, what a good world we live in! How good and beautiful! How young it is, too, with nothing really rotten or age-worn in it!" (pp. 213–214). He is wrong: it is Phoebe, standing by his side at that time, who is the source of this bliss. He discovers that secret of the heart when he is rescued from despair the instant Phoebe's presence is made real to him by the touch of her hand. What was true for Clifford is now true for Holgrave: "Holding her hand, you felt something; a tender something; a substance, and a warm one; and so long as you should feel its grasp, soft as it was, you might be certain that your place was good in the whole sympathetic chain of human nature. The world was no longer a delusion" (p. 141). The rupture is repaired; being reunited with Phoebe is the remedy for his alienation from the sympathetic chain of humanity. Holgrave neither must face alone the "rude struggle of man with man" nor is he compelled to tear down all that is "really rotten and age-worn" because with Phoebe it is "a good world that we live in!" (pp. 213–214).[16] The revolution in his feelings is so powerful and so immediately brought about by Phoebe's presence that the connection is now undeniable: "But Phoebe, you crossed the threshold; and hope, warmth and joy, came with you! The black moment became at once a blissful one. It must not pass without the spoken word. I love you!" (Vol. 2, p. 306). The defenses that had kept him self-contained dissolve in the refulgent feelings of love, and he allows himself to yield, in utter trusting dependence, to Phoebe: "You are my only possibility of happiness! … I have no faith in it, except as you bestow it on me!" (Vol. 2, p. 306). Although sin and guilt are universal, since they are found "in the depth of every heart" (Vol. 9, p. 306), they can be mediated and made bearable through the office of love. In his interchange in the garden with Phoebe, Holgrave anticipates this transformative experience; he has here found abundant reparation for his sudden loss of innocence: "Our first youth is of no value; for we are never conscious of it, until after it is gone. But sometimes … there comes a sense of second youth, gushing out of the heart's joy at being in love.… In some cases, the two states come, almost simultaneously, and mingle the sadness and the rapture in one mysterious emotion" (p. 215). The incomparably beautiful culmination of the romance, when the black moment becomes blissful, expresses this truth.

The last thing that Holgrave does before Phoebe appears is take a daguerreotype of Jaffrey's form, a sort of death mask. He has had to confront Death; with the daguerreotype, Holgrave, as artist, transforms traumatic experience into a work of art. He shows Phoebe the image of Jaffrey to spare her the trauma of actually seeing his dead body. In this way, art, like love, mediates and makes bearable the most painful aspects of life and death. There is no reason to believe that Holgrave will not continue to fulfill his promise as a visual artist and as a writer and that he will not be, as Baym predicts, "the failure of the artist-hero." His union with Phoebe may demotivate efforts at radical reform, but it does not corrupt his artistic nature; these endeavors arise from different internal sources. If anything, Phoebe will offer restoratives from the strenuous demands of artistic creativity: "[A]t his highest elevation, the poets need no intercourse; but he finds it dreary to descend, and be a stranger" (p. 141). Hawthorne knew of what he spoke: *The Scarlet Letter* and the three romances that followed it, including, of course, *The House of the Seven Gables*, mark a distinctive maturation in his fiction, and all were written during his marriage to Sophia Peabody.

Holgrave foresees a modification in his hitherto-radical social philosophy as a means to reassure Phoebe, who is concerned that, in her conventionality, she will "have not scope enough to make you happy" (p. 306); he tells her, "The world owes all its onward impulse to men ill at ease. The happy man inevitably confines himself within ancient limits" (pp. 306–307). This is a reprise of the sentiment he expressed in the garden under the influence of romantic enchantment: "Moonlight, and the sentiment in man's heart, responsive to it, is the greatest of renovators and reformers. And all other reform and renovation, I suppose, will prove no better than moonshine!" (p. 214). It is love that transforms reality. Holgrave has come to the wisdom that is expressed at the end of "Earth's Holocaust:" "Purify that inner sphere; and the many shapes of evil that haunt the outward, and which now seem almost our only realities, will turn to shadowy phantoms, and vanish of their own accord" (Vol. 10, p. 404). Under love's dispensation, the compulsions pertaining to the House of the Seven Gables, both attractions and repulsions, "vanish of their own accord," as it were, and the House loses its vast symbolic power. The Judge's country house will be lived in "for the present" (p. 314); it need not be held by its new occupants as a status of wealth and privilege. Holgrave remains true to his conscience because the idea of settling in a house, "planting a family," now that he is with Phoebe and her relatives, has "at a moment's warning … establish[ed] its right to hold its ground" (p. 177). Neither is it likely, because he now sees the virtues of possessing a house of his own, that he cannot fulfill his potential as "the champion of some practicable cause" (p. 181). Holgrave's idealism, "which a young man had better never have been born, than not to have" (p. 179), may be tempered, but he remains an intelligent, sensitive man of integrity and an accomplished artist. And, if he says "Ah, Phoebe, I told you how it would be! … You find me a conservative already!" with "a half-melancholy laugh" (p. 315), it speaks for a wistful backward glance at the passing of youthful fantasy and not, as Baym suggests, the expression of a "brooding melancholy man" (p. 95) or of Von Abele's "settled and weary conservative" (p. 59). It is, after all, a laugh. The narrator employs precisely the same description to Phoebe's pensive comment: "'Ah, poor me!' she added, with a half-melancholy laugh, 'I shall never be so merry as before I knew Cousin Hepzibah and poor Cousin Clifford'" (p. 214).

Other significant changes radiate from Holgrave's transformation. In the past, the Maules, always marginal, have not participated in the life of their community. Making common cause with Phoebe and her family, Holgrave is no longer an isolate on the fringe of society. He will lend his talents and energies to sustaining a multigenerational community bound by love and respect. Clifford and Hepzibah will need to be sustained and protected; their protracted and painful isolation in prison and in the House is ended. Uncle Venner, who inhabits "the very lowest point of the social scale" (p. 155), will be afforded the status of a venerated elder, as well as refuge from what would have been the relegation to a poor house. As for the future, if Holgrave and Phoebe's successful cultivation of the House's garden is any sign, there will soon be another generation to be nurtured. The realm of community power has been presided over by Jaffrey Pyncheon; Richard H. Millington (1992) suggests that, in its social vision, *The House of the Seven Gables* attempts "to build an alternate cultural consensus" (p. 130) that can "transform that community center in the very act of occupying it" (p. 106). In occupying Jaffrey's "country-seat," Holgrave, Phoebe et al. will be in a position, literally and figuratively, to work toward this end. In a wonderful stroke of irony, this patchwork gathering of individuals into an inclusive community gives substance in its way to Holgrave's idealistic vision that, in "this very now, there are harbingers abroad of a golden era, to be accomplished in his own life time" (p. 179).[17]

Holgrave's transformation has its moral aspect, too. In his agitation, Holgrave voices to Phoebe deep concern about what will happen to Clifford when Jaffrey's body is discovered: "But Clifford! ... Clifford and Hepzibah! We must consider what is best to be done in their behalf .... How miserably unfortunate!" (p. 303). Holgrave now wants to *do*, not just to *look*. He finally gives a palpable answer to Phoebe's inquiry: "How is it possible to see people in distress, without desiring, more than anything else, to help and comfort them?" (p. 217). In doing so, he passes a last test of character and is now worthy of Phoebe. His crisis has wrought a moral enlightenment, and with it a form of *caritas*, that renders him "more like a christian and a human being" (p. 217).[18]

F. O. Matthiessen's (1941) commentary on the end of the romance has been influential for several generations of literary critics: "Yet in the poetic justice of bestowing opulence on all those who had previously been deprived of it by the Judge, Hawthorne overlooked the fact that he was sowing all over again the same seeds of evil" (p. 332). The vantage offered by this psychological study allows me to suggest a different judgment. Although opulence may sow the seeds of evil, those seeds need not be cultivated. It is doubtful that, as portrayed in all their humanity, these sterling individuals, so conditioned by adversity and poverty, would have any inclination to join company with avaricious abusers of wealth and power, such as Jaffrey, even though they dwell in his elegant house. One would have to overlook the emotional wisdom of *The House of the Seven Gables* to believe that will be their fate. It is true that the future is uncertain and there is always the possibility of moral failings. Millington is correct that "[b]oth lovers have a strikingly clear-eyed sense of the difficulties that will attend their union" (p. 148). However, there is much hope in a new generation represented by the likes of Holgrave and Phoebe, upon whom will fall the hard work of molding the granite substance of the earth into usable forms. For them, at least, that lifelong task will be informed by the tragedies of the past and the indelible transformations that misfortune has wrought upon their deepest being.

Mimosa Stephenson's illuminating thesis that both tragedy and comedy inhere in every aspect of *The House of the Seven Gables* also has relevance for a different understanding of the romance's providential ending. Hawthorne never overlooked the tragic potential in all things human. Instead, the romance's conclusion bears witness to "the fiercer, deeper, and more tragic power of laughter" (p. 164). Through Jaffrey's death, tragedy has been averted, and the romance's ending, with its resonances of Greek and divine comedy, celebrates the joyous prospect that, with evil annulled, all goodness is possible and happiness attainable.

The black moment had become at once a blissful one.

Notes

1. The antitheses that Holgrave encompasses are but a few of many examples of the literary device that Mimosa Stephenson (2013) elucidates in her outstanding essay "Humor as Antithesis in *The House of the Seven Gables*."
2. Moreover, by ignoring the contribution of Holgrave's conscious processing of his experience during his vigil with the Judge's corpse and by focusing, instead, solely on unconscious contents, Crews falls prey to a temptation that gave the early crop of psychoanalytic interpretations of literary works a bad name, namely, to view a character's manifestation of psychic agency entirely as a symptom of neurosis. Crews's Oedipal interpretation of the scene lacks explanatory power and impoverishes rather than enriches an understanding of Holgrave's transformation. In his essay, "Freud and Literature," Lionel Trilling (1950) levels a devastating critique at the traditional Freudian mode of literary interpretation from which, it might be said, it has never fully recovered.
3. Hawthorne had closely read the works of his literary forbear, James Fenimore Cooper; there are many parallels between *The House of the Seven Gables* and *The Pioneers*, published in 1823. Like Holgrave, the hero of *The Pioneers*, Edward Oliver, in his return to Judge Templeton's estate, carries with him a secret resentment over hereditary injustice involving ancestral property. The novel concludes in a reconciliation between the two families with the marriage of Oliver to Elizabeth Templeton. For all his condescension toward Hawthorne, in *Little Dorritt* (1855), Charles Dickens appears to have borrowed generously from plot and thematic elements in *The House of the Seven Gables*. The secret of the Clennam family's wrongful appropriation of the fortune belonging to the Dorritts is revealed at the novel's conclusion, which also celebrates the rapprochement of the two families in the marriage of Little Dorritt to Arthur Clennam. The pathetic William Dorritt's imprisonment and Little Dorritt's devotion to him resonates with Clifford's incarceration and Phoebe's ministrations; and in reversals of fortune, both the elder Dorritt and Clifford become wealthy. For other points of similarity, see Leavis (1991).
4. Holgrave joins the pantheon of Hawthorne voyeurs: Chillingworth (*The Scarlet Letter*), Coverdale (*The Blithedale Romance*), and The Model (*The Marble Faun*).
5. See my "'There is nothing but love here.'"
6. Holgrave's love for Phoebe is an instance of Pascal's wisdom: *le coeur a ses raison que la raison ne connaît point* (the heart has its reasons that reason knows nothing of).
7. Holgrave's sketch of Matthew Maule closely resembles that of the narrator's regarding the daguerreotypist's less seemly side: "[W]hat worked most to the young carpenter's disadvantage, was, first, the reserve and sternness of

his natural disposition . . . and the suspicion of his holding heretical tenets in matters of religion and polity" (p. 190). At various points, Holgrave's reserve, sternness, and heretical tenets are alluded to.

8. Similarly, Holgrave refers to himself to Phoebe as "[a] mere observer . . . (who never [has] any intuitions, and am, at best, only subtile and acute)" (p. 179).
9. Note the similarity to the description of Old Moodie at Zenobia's funeral in *The Blithedale Romance*: "Nearest the dead walked an old man in deep mourning, his face mostly concealed in a white handkerchief, and with Priscilla leaning on his arm" (Hawthorne, 1962, Vol. 3, p. 239). In gratuitously stripping Zenobia of the entirety of her fortune in favor of Priscilla, Old Moodie also meant to humble her in her pride; instead, he provokes her suicide.
10. Nor could Jaffrey Pyncheon have both a loving wife and a slave. His subjugation of his young bride led to her early death: "[T]he lady got her death-blow in the honey-moon, and never smiled again, because her husband compelled her to serve him with coffee, every morning, at his bedside, in token of fealty to her liege-lord and master" (p. 123).
11. Of course, Phoebe is no Alice: she is a poor working girl and has no aristocratic pretensions; moreover, she is respectful and somewhat deferential toward Holgrave, certainly not condescending.
12. In his allegorical journey, Holgrave finds himself in Bunyan's Slough of Despond.
13. Both the narrator's and Holgrave's experience of the corpse evolve from the personal to the allegorical; Magnus Ullén's (2004) insight regarding allegory as a mode of conceptualizing the "distance between an experience felt and an experience expressed, between content and form" has particular relevance to this point in the narrative. I agree with him that, in his allegorical invention, Hawthorne "invite[s] us to explicate their truths by establishing their meaning" (p. 91).
14. Hawthorne eschews the narration of his characters' profound psychological transformations, and there are important instances in each romance. An analysis of a similar narrative gap regarding Dimmesdale's transformation in *The Scarlet Letter* is found in Chapter Two, "'*That self was gone!*'" Hester Prynne's decision to return to Boston falls in a narrative silence that envelopes her at the moment of Dimmesdale's death on the scaffold. In *The Blithedale Romance*, Zenobia's contemplation and enactment of suicide occur when the narrator, Coverdale, is asleep. Shlomith Rimmon-Kenan (1977) presents a masterful analysis of narrative gaps in *The Concept of Ambiguity* (pp. 45–51).
15. Death is the great instructor in all Hawthorne romances. Dimmesdale's death on the scaffold in *The Scarlet Letter* inspires moral transformations in those who witnessed it: Pearl, Chillingworth, and Hester. Coverdale's memoir, which is the substance of *The Blithedale Romance*, is an act of mourning for Zenobia's death, and is analyzed in Chapter Four. In *The Marble Faun*, the murder of the Model determines the subsequent fate of all the characters, which is the subject of Chapter Five, "'The tragic dignity of their hour of crime.'"
16. Edward A. Dryden (1971) points out the similarity between the change in Holgrave's worldview wrought by his love for Phoebe and Hawthorne's description, recorded in *The American Notebooks*, of the transformation of his worldview consequent to his marriage to Sophia: "The fight with the world—the struggle of a man among men—the agony of the universal

effort to wrench the means of life from a host of greedy competitors—all this seems like a dream to me. My business is merely to live and to enjoy; and whatever is essential to life and enjoyment will come as naturally as the dew from the Heavens" (p. 313).

17. Hawthorne will explore the communitarian endeavor in his next novel, *The Blithedale Romance*. Alas, without the transformation of the human heart as its foundation, the effort is destined to failure.
18. Holgrave's moral enlightenment, with its distinctly Christian coloring, is a facet of what Gatta (1978) insightfully traces as *The House of the Seven Gables*'s "underground stream of sacred history progressing toward final apocalyptic fulfillment," which reaches its climax with the alliance of Holgrave and Phoebe and represents "the cosmic marriage celebrated in the Book of Revelation" (p. 46).

References

Baym, N. (1970). The Failure of the Artist-Hero. *The Journal of English and German Philology, 69.*

Chodorow, N. J. (1999). *The Power of Feelings.* New Haven: Princeton.

Cooper, J. (1823). *The Pioneers.* Oxford: Oxford University Press.

Crews, F. (1996). *The Sins of the Father: Hawthorne's Psychological Themes.* New York: Oxford University Press.

Diamond, D. (2002). "There is nothing but love here": Toward a Recovery from Massive Psychic Trauma in *The House of the Seven Gables. Nathaniel Hawthorne Review*, *28*, 61–68.

Dryden, E. (1971). Hawthorne's Castle in the Air: Form and Theme in *The House of the Seven Gables. ELH*, *38*(2), 294–317.

Gatta, J. Jr. (1978). Progress and Providence in *The House of the Seven Gables. American Literature*, *38*(2), 37–48.

Hawthorne, N. (1962a). *The Blithedale Romance.* In W. Charvat (Ed.), *The Centenary Edition of the Works of Nathaniel Hawthorne* (Vol. 3). Columbus: Ohio State University Press.

Hawthorne, N. (1962b). *The House of the Seven Gables.* In W. Charvat (Ed.), *The Centenary Edition of the Works of Nathaniel Hawthorne* (Vol. 2). Columbus: Ohio University State Press.

Hawthorne, N. (1962c). *The Marble Faun.* In W. Charvat (Ed.), *The Centenary Edition of the Works of Nathaniel Hawthorne* (Vol. 4). Columbus: Ohio State University Press.

Hawthorne, N. (1962d). *The Scarlet Letter.* In W. Charvat (Ed.), *The Centenary Edition of the Works of Nathaniel Hawthorne* (Vol. 1). Columbus: Ohio State University Press.

Hawthorne, N. (1974a). The Hall of Fantasy. In W. Charvat (Ed.), *The Centenary Edition of the Works of Nathaniel Hawthorne* (Vol. 10). Columbus: Ohio State University Press.

Hawthorne, N. (1974b). The Haunted Mind. In *The Centenary Editions of the Works of Nathaniel Hawthorne* (Vol. 9). Columbus: Ohio University State Press.

Keegan, P. (2017). From Shtetl to Boulevard. *The London Review of Books, 39.*

Leavis, L. (1991). Dickens and Hawthorne: *Little Dorritt* and *The House of the Seven Gables. English Studies*, *72*(5), 414–420.

Matthiessen, F. O. (1941). *American Renaissance: Art and Expression in the Age of Emerson and Whitman*. New York: Oxford University Press.
Millington, R. H. (1992). *Practicing Romance: Narrative Form and Cultural Engagement in Hawthorne's Fiction*. Princeton: Princeton University Press.
Perry, D. (2014). The 'Strangely Mingled Elements' of *The House of the Seven Gables*: The Fairy-Tale Art of Telling the Truth. *Nathaniel Hawthorne Society Conference*. North Adams, MA.
Rimmon-Kenan, S. (1977). *The Concept of Ambiguity–the Example of James*. Chicago: University of Chicago Press.
Stephenson, M. (2013). Humor as Antithesis in *The House of the Seven Gables*. *Nathaniel Hawthorne Review*, *39*(2), 105–25.
Trilling, L. (1950). Freud and Literature. In *The Liberal Imagination: Essays on Literature and Society* (pp. 34–57). New York: Viking.
Ullén, M. (2004). *The Half-Vanished Structure: Hawthorne's Allegorical Dialectics*. Bern: Peter Lang.
Von Abele, R. (1955). *The Death of the Artist: A Study of Hawthorne's Disintegration*. Nijhoff.
Yoder, R. (1974). Transcendental Conservatism and *The House of the Seven Gables*. *The Georgia Review*, *28*(1), 33–51.

4 Zenobia's Suicide in *The Blithedale Romance:* "But, all this while, we have been standing by Zenobia's grave"

Zenobia's suicide is the defining act around which *The Blithedale Romance* is constellated: all parts of the narrative converge toward it and radiate from it. The night of the first gathering at Blithedale, Zenobia's death is augured when "the black shadow of the only cloud in heaven ... swept across our door-step. How cold an Arcadia was this!" (Hawthorne, 1962, Vol. 3, p. 38). More pointedly, at the end of Coverdale's first day at Blithedale, Zenobia prefigures her fate when, in a poetical parody, she addresses him:

> you had better turn the affair into a ballad. It is a grand subject ... The storm, the startling knock at the door, the entrance of the sable knight Hollingsworth and this shadowy snow-maiden, who, precisely at the stroke of midnight, shall melt away at my feet, into a pool of ice-cold water, and give me my death with a pair of wet slippers! (p. 33).

And so, more it less, it comes to be: five months later, Zenobia's drowned body is recovered from the river near midnight after she had been given her death, in part, by Priscilla's usurpation of her love and fortune. The optimism of the first phase of the Blithedale enterprise, reflected in the light-hearted tone of Zenobia's prediction, turns to dark portent as the central characters become entangled in an "inextricable knot" (p. 98). Coverdale is correct to worry that, "between Zenobia's passionate force and his [Hollingsworth's] dark, self-delusive egotism" might "develop itself in some sufficiently tragic catastrophe" (p. 79). In the interchange with Coverdale immediately before she commits suicide, Zenobia wryly comments about her situation: "It is genuine tragedy, is it not?" (p. 223). It is: Hawthorne's Zenobia is a tragic heroine who is elevated by nobility, generosity of spirit, creative intelligence, and passionate beauty. Despite flaws and vulnerabilities which contribute to her undoing, she resists a society whose rules are set against her as a woman but succumbs when its harsh, narrow judgments converge with destructive forces arising from her past which she can no longer flee.

At the end of the romance, twelve years after her death, Coverdale avers, "But, all this while, we have been standing by Zenobia's grave" (p. 243). This, and not the fatuous and thinly-concealed love that he held for Priscilla, is the crucial secret that he has kept from the reader. In light of this assertion, the entire narrative, conceived as it is from such a vantage, needs to be re-interpreted as an extended series of associations to Zenobia's death. At the end, when Coverdale glimpses a broken Hollingsworth, slavishly supported by Priscilla's "puny weakness" (p. 224), and as he reflects on his own non-productive life in the intervening years, it is apparent that all three have been suspended in a state of prolonged grief: the cloud of Zenobia's death has cast its black shadow over all their prospects. The "ballad" that Coverdale does eventually write can be interpreted as an act of mourning for Zenobia. Coverdale has finally satisfied her exhortation, "But, Mr. Coverdale, by all means, write this ballad, and put your soul's ache into it, and turn your sympathy to good account, as other poets do, and as poets must, unless they choose to give us glittering icicles instead of lines of fire" (p. 224). In his concluding "confession," Coverdale states: "As for poetry, I have given it up" (p. 246), but the reader must not be misled by his proclivity to "exaggerate my own defects" (p. 247): by transforming his memoirs into *The Blithedale Romance*, Coverdale has turned from poet to romancer, and has written a masterpiece.

Despite its centrality in the novel, Zenobia's suicide eludes facile comprehension, even by those who knew her well. The characters express disbelief that her situation warranted self-destruction. Silas Foster exclaims, "What on earth should the young woman do that for?...There's some mistake about this, I tell you!" (pp. 230–231). Westervelt is scornful: "It was an idle thing –a foolish thing—for Zenobia to do! ... She was the last woman in the world to whom death could have been necessary" (p. 239). He adds, "Love had failed her, you say! Had it never failed her before? Yet she survived and loved again – possibly not once alone, nor twice either. And now to drown herself for yonder dreamy philanthropist!" (p. 240). Coverdale is more sympathetic to her plight and states: "If any crisis could justify this sad wrong she offered to herself, it was surely that in which she stood. Everything had failed her –prosperity in the world's sense, for her opulence was gone –the heart's prosperity, in love" (p. 239). However, he remains perplexed "that a woman of Zenobia's diverse capacity should have fancied herself irretrievably defeated on the broad battle-field of life, and with no refuge, save to fall on her own sword, merely because Love had gone against her" (p. 241). The words "fancied" and "merely" indicate a failure to fathom the devastation wrought by Hollingsworth's separating himself from her which leaves her feeling "poor, despised, rejected" (p. 227).[1]

What Coverdale does not appreciate at that time is that Zenobia experiences the rejection as broader than that of one particular man. She is on trial by a "secret tribunal [of men]" which "chances to be the only judgment-seat that a true woman stands in awe of, and that any verdict short of acquittal is equivalent to a death sentence!" (p. 215). It is her womanhood which is being judged. Hollingsworth attempts to contradict this expansive conclusion: "True; I have already judged you, but not on the world's part, —neither do I pretend to pass a sentence!" (p. 215). Unchanged in her conviction, Zenobia will soon execute what she considers to be the tribunal's death sentence.

The depth of Zenobia's feelings of rejection is a catalyst to her suicide and will be the subject of this essay's inquiry. Critics, of course, have sought to make sense of Zenobia's action. Emphasizing that Hollingsworth's judgment of her is issued as if by a stern Puritan magistrate, Nina Baym (1968) sympathizes with the magnitude of the rejection: "As a life force, she has been put down; as a woman, she has been denied a place in the world administered by men. She kills herself, as she must" (pp. 567–568). Elizabeth Dill (2011) underscores the idealistic aspects of Zenobia's suicide which she interprets as "part of a sentimental gesture of self-sacrifice to the ideals Blithedale represents" (p. 66); this view, although it takes into account Zenobia's altruism, is hard to reconcile with her parting sentiment that Blilthedale was "a foolish dream" (Hawthorne, 1962, Vol. 3, p. 227). Terence J. Matheson (1976) considers that Zenobia is punished by conscience: she destroys herself "when the full truth of herself and the extent of her previous self-deception fully dawns on her" (p. 117). Whether a consequence of misogyny, idealism, or conscience, these critics approach Zenobia's suicide as a matter with gravitas.

For the most part, however, and unlike Hester's plight in *The Scarlet Letter*, Zenobia's arouses little empathy among most critics. What they repeatedly emphasize, and as a critical judgment, is the dramatic quality of her suicide. William L. Hedges (1960) contends that Zenobia's presence at Blithdedale is a ploy meant to "use liberal movements only as a stage on which to give her essentially theatrical personality room to act" (p. 308). Frederick Crews (1966), who describes Zenobia as a "brash and busomy feminist," (p. 202) considers her farewell to Coverdale "somewhat histrionic" (p. 207). Ffrangeon Lewis (1992) takes this characterization further in judging that Zenobia's "final gesture is indeed an eloquent piece of self-conscious self-dramatization" (p. 78). Leo B. Levy (1968) considers her suicide to be "her acquiescence to the image of the wronged village girl which she seizes in order to dramatize her rejections by Hollingsworth" (p. 7). John N. Miller (2000) concurs that in her "'tragic' role', Zenobia gives herself the opportunity to 'play' a love-crazed Ophelia and submit herself to death by drowning" (p. 15). Nor does Hawthorne escape criticism for having created an ending that, in Bill Christophersen's (1982) judgment, "lacks dramatic necessity… Zenobia's death remains melodrama and *not* tragedy" (p. 89). The interpretation of Zenobia's suicide as an enactment of a piece of drama for effect, rather than an authentic expression of her being, impoverishes the range of its meanings that I believe Hawthorne would have us contemplate. All the more is Zenobia's status as a tragic figure negated by those critics who go so far as to deny that she, in fact, committed suicide. John Harmon McElroy and Edward L. McDonald (1982) find "evidence" that is "considerable and seems conclusive" that Coverdale murdered her (p. 89). As accomplished a Hawthorne critic as Michael J. Colarcurcio (2008) takes this theory sufficiently seriously to dignify it with mention on a par with that of Zenobia's death being by suicide: "If Coverdale kills her, it is because her fatal attraction to Hollingsworth has insulted his own less aggressive manhood. If she kills herself it is because Hollingsworth is incorrigibly attracted to the pliant Priscilla" (p. 22).[2] Apart from the overwhelming evidence in the text against this notion and, given the definitively passive cast to Coverdale's psychology, its implausibility, such a reading robs Zenobia of the power of her action and subverts Hawthorne's moral purpose by transforming the romance's tragic conclusion into a farce. Zenobia issues cautionary wisdom to the critics who deny her serious purpose: "There can be no truer test of the noble and heroic, in any individual, than the degree he possesses the faculty of distinguishing heroism from absurdity" (Vol. 3, p.166).

During his interchange with Westervelt at Zenobia's funeral, Coverdale searches for Zenobia's motivation beyond the rupture with Hollingsworth: "And there was a secret burthen on her, the nature of which is best known to you" (p. 239). Coverdale is alluding to Zenobia's hitherto cryptic relationship with Westervelt: while in his "hermitage," he overhears Zenobia's interchange with Westervelt in which she rails against the "miserable bond" that "will strangle me at last!" (p. 104). Undoubtedly her life being "hopelessly entangled with a villain's" (p. 225) magnifies a desperate need for release from this bondage. However, I would suggest that there is another and largely unappreciated burden on Zenobia, namely, the recent discovery that her father is alive in the person of Old Moodie. In transferring all her wealth to Priscilla, he is responsible for her abrupt fall from prosperity to poverty which is linked to Hollingsworth's severing of his attachment to her. There is no narration of Zenobia's discovery of this momentous secret, but we gauge its impact in her allusion to her father when, perhaps already having decided her fate, she kisses Priscilla farewell, "not lovingly; for a sense of fatal harm received through her, seemed to be lurking in Zenobia's heart" (pp. 219–220). Zenobia then says to Priscilla, "We had one father! You knew it from the first; I, but a little while –else some things, that have chanced, might have been spared you" (p. 220). It is her father who, through Priscilla, inflicts "fatal harm" upon her.

Old Moodie, in convening his own private "secret tribunal" by which he judges and condemns Zenobia's behavior toward Priscilla, whom he has kept from knowing is her half-sister, and in gratuitously stripping her of the entirety of her fortune because he is not pleased by what he witnesses in this family drama of his own creation, is perhaps the most pernicious character in Hawthorne's oeuvre. Coverdale aptly refers to him as "this deplorable Old Moodie" (p. 88). Zenobia is, after all, his daughter, and a thoroughly admirable young woman, who has never done him any harm. As fate would have it, his action against her, which causes loss of love and material support, constitutes a repetition of the childhood traumata she also suffered at his hands. Old Moodie had wasted the family fortune, turned criminal, and then abandoned her and her mother who died of shame and grief. Zenobia's past has overtaken her attempts at a new life at Blithedale and Old Moodie is again the agent of irreparable loss.

The vulnerabilities that arise from her childhood color her life and gather to oppress her final days. Freud emphasized the continuity of psychic life:

conflicts and traumata arising in childhood are recorded in the unconscious where they exert influence throughout life. Hawthorne anticipates Freud's conception of the dynamic unconscious in his early sketch, "The Haunted Mind" (1835): "In the depths of every heart, there is a tomb and a dungeon, though the lights, the music, the revelry above may cause us to forget their existence, and the buried ones, or prisoners whom they hide. But sometimes, and oftenest at midnight, those dark receptacles are flung wide open" (Vol. 9, p. 306). With the loss of fortune and prospects for love, the "lights, music and revelry" of Zenobia's opulent manner dissipate and she is brought to remember the "buried ones" who then emerge from her haunted mind with staggering force. The narrator captures the terrible moment when, after Hollingsworth finally departs with Priscilla:

> ...she began slowly to sink down. It was as if a great, invisible, irresistible weight were pressing her to the earth. Settling upon her knees, she leaned her forehead against the rock, and sobbed convulsively; dry sobs, they seemed to be, such as have nothing to do with tears (p. 221).

I will begin by generating a portrait of Zenobia as she appeared in her splendor to Coverdale and others during the apparently care-free beginnings of the Blithedale endeavor. From this lofty elevation, we can appreciate the tragedy of her eventual fall. The story of her childhood, which is elicited from Old Moodie by Coverdale, is recorded in Chapter XXII, "Fauntleroy," and will serve as the basis for a psychoanalytically informed narrative of Zenobia's life before and at Blithedale, one which sets the foundation for interpreting her suicide.

In order to contextualize this narrative, I will draw on Nancy Chodorow's (1999) contrast between psychoanalytic epistemology and that of other humanistic disciplines. She writes: "Because psychological meaning is constitutive of internal and external perceptions and experiences from childhood on, the past is always drawn into the present" (p. 60). Chodorow considers psychoanalysis "first and foremost an account and theory of personal meaning" (p. 129), and its method is to unravel "the particularistic uniqueness of each individual psyche and life history" (p. 2). In its systematic consideration of "the power of feelings," which is the pithy title that Chodorow has given to her thought-provoking book, psychoanalysis distinguishes itself from other interpretive frameworks such as linguistic, historicist and feminist, to name a few.[3] The narrative that I have constructed follows the vicissitudes of the determinative power of feelings in a contextual continuum from Zenobia's childhood to her crisis at Blithedale; in so doing, I seek to contribute to an understanding of the psychological underpinnings of her ultimate act. Behavior is always over-determined, but suicide cries out for illumination of its psychological motivations.

Joel Pfister (1991) is concerned that: "Psychoanalysis tends to foreclose our consideration of social and historical processes" (p. 86). The analysis that follows does not mean to foreclose other perspectives but, by giving expression to a distinctive psychoanalytic voice, to complement them, and to invite response in the ongoing critical conversation about Zenobia and *The Blithedale Romance.*

Zenobia and Coverdale

It is hardly an exaggeration to consider Zenobia, as portrayed by so exacting an observer as Coverdale, one of the most outstanding women in American literature. She was a well-known icon in Boston's reformist intellectual circles and was addressed by her intimates by her nom de plume, "Zenobia," an appellation that suggests resonances between the nobility of her character, which is repeatedly emphasized by the narrator, and that of her namesake, the Palmyrean Queen, Zenobia.[4] In Coverdale's informed estimation, she had a "fine intellect" (p. 15) which was employed in writing essays, including feminist "tracts in defense of the sex" (p. 33) and short fiction which was published in local journals. Coverdale may not have been impressed with her as a writer, but apparently the editors of those periodicals were. Her strength, as Zenobia admits, was in oratory. She was in the vanguard of feminism, decrying the suppression of women's voices in public discourse, and had won recognition as a compelling lecturer on the rights of women. She possessed a theatrical flare and her dramatic readings of Shakespeare at Blithedale, performed, in Coverdale's considered opinion, with "depth of tragic power, or breadth of comic effect" (p. 106) won the audience's admiration. In the execution of *tableaux vivants*, she demonstrated unusual abilities in the visual arts as well as a knowledge of the Old Masters. The aesthetics of her opulent Boston apartment, certainly of her own design, overwhelmed Coverdale's sensibility, as did her ability to dress an asthenic Priscilla to startling advantage. In her drawing-room, Coverdale discovered that she was an accomplished pianist. Zenobia's literary tastes were sophisticated and included an appreciation of George Sand, the socially daring French novelist and feminist with whom she undoubtedly identified, and whose novels she provided to Coverdale during his convalescence.[5] From their first encounter at Blithedale, Zenobia encouraged Coverdale to continue to write poetry and we cannot doubt the sincerity of her appreciation, nor the headiness of her praise of it, expressed in her gracious first greeting: "I have long wished to know you, Mr. Coverdale, and to thank you for your beautiful poetry, some of which I have learned by heart;–or, rather, it has stolen into my memory" (p. 14). She was generous in her affluence, as she had provided "liberal pecuniary aid" (p. 177) to the Blithedale enterprise. Nor was she an armchair egalitarian; although she maintained an in-town dwelling, she committed herself in deed to a community which "meant to lessen the laboring man's great burthen of toil" (p. 19). As a social reformer, not unlike Holgrave in *The House of the Seven Gables,* she was determinedly radical. Coverdale remarks on "the hardihood of her philosophy; she made no scruple of oversetting all human institutions, and scattering them as with a breeze of her fan" (p. 44). She brought reform from theory into practice in organizing the Blithedale work schema; although equality of the sexes in that regard was a goal, she was willing to do her share of traditional woman's chores during a period of transition.[6] She never claimed leadership but authority was afforded to her because of her competence and commanding personality. Her acceptance of Priscilla the first night of her appearance ensured the peculiar young woman's acceptance by the community. And in the final masquerade, the community fittingly crowned her Queen Zenobia. With her many endowments and accomplishments, Zenobia's resemblance to Hawthorne's interlocutor and one-time friend, Margaret Fuller, has often been commented on in the critical literature.[7] Coverdale refers to Fuller as "one of the most gifted women of the age" (p. 51); I believe that within the world of *The Blithedale Romance*, the same can be said of Zenobia.

I dwell on Zenobia's qualities that have no direct relation to her striking physical appearance. Zenobia is aware of the mutability of physical attractiveness. In response to Coverdale's lyrical advocacy of governance by a woman ruler, she incisively queries: "Yes; if she were young and beautiful...But how if she were sixty and a fright?" (p. 121). That said, Coverdale describes Zenobia as "truly a magnificent woman" (p. 44) with an irresistible physical allure. He admires the "bounteous nature of this beautiful woman" (p. 21) who was "womanliness incarnated" (p. 44). She talked with "so much vivacity" (p. 44) and with an "inimitable voice" (p. 107) which was "fine, frank, mellow" (p. 14). Her laugh was "delectable to hear" (p. 16); her hand was "very soft and warm" (p. 14); and her hair, "dark, glossy, and of singular abundance" (p. 15). There was a "queenliness of her presence" (p. 44) as she carried herself with "pride and pomp" (p. 15). The superlative qualities of Zenobia's physical being are interwoven with those of her noble character: "that noble and beautiful motion which characterized her as much as any other personal charm" was "the result and expression of the whole being... responsive to something in the character" (p. 155). Moreover she possessed "the sweet, liberal, but womanly frankness of a noble and generous disposition" (p. 47). In a different mood, she could demonstrate a "free, careless, generous mode of expression" (p. 17) and a capacity for exuberantly sardonic humor.

Given his acute aesthetic sensibility, we have no compelling reason to question Coverdale's characterization of Zenobia's appearance. However, the reader must exercise caution regarding his impressions of her sexuality *per se*, which tend to reveal more about him than necessarily about her. Coverdale assigns responsibility for his sexual arousal to a force outside himself, as he exclaims to Hollingsworth: "Zenobia is an enchantress!" (p. 45). In response to her humorous allusion to the garb of the Garden of Eden, Coverdale "irresistibly" (p. 17) imagines Zenobia's "fine, perfectly developed figure" (p. 17) standing naked before his eyes. The fantasy has the force of reality: "Behold, here is a woman!" (p. 17). Coverdale's arousal is urgent and sufficiently uncomfortable as to necessitate defenses against it. With no knowledge of her past, and while accusing himself of "masculine grossness —a sin of wicked interpretation" (p. 47), he nonetheless comes to the conclusion that Zenobia is sexually experienced, that "the gates of mystery" (p. 47) for her have been "thrown wide" (p. 47). In Coverdale's mind, even a suspicion to this effect, and colored by his own desire, is sufficient evidence for his own "secret tribunal" to return a harsh judgment that she is guilty of having already "given herself away" (p. 48) and thereby to have "defrauded" (p. 48) a bachelor such as himself. Coverdale's psyche propels him down the slippery slope of unconscious defenses against his sexual desire: by employing the mechanism of projective identification, he flings his own wishes for sexual gratification onto Zenobia, then condemns her for what he should consider his own erotic crime. Finally, the anxiety aroused by the conflict over his sexual urges leads to a phobic avoidance of the object of desire: "The riddle made me so nervous, however, in my sensitive condition of mind and body, that I most ungratefully began to wish that she would let me alone" (p. 48). Lowe (2017) comments: "As Coverdale does again and again when met with the specter of actual sexuality, he runs away" (p. 67). Whether or not Zenobia has had sexual experience is not the point, but the way that Coverdale arrives at his conviction about the matter is instructive as it gives weight to Zenobia's later accusation that Coverdale's "cold-blooded criticism [is] founded on a shallow interpretation of half-perceptions" (Hawthorne, 1962, Vol. 3, p. 170).

It is an impressive irony that Coverdale, who boasts that regarding his friends he endeavors "by generous sympathies, by delicate intuitions, by taking note of things too slight for record, and by bringing my human spirit into manifold accordance with the companions whom God assigned me – to learn the secret which was hidden even from themselves," (p. 160) keeps hidden from himself the promptings of his heart. The exultant descriptions of Zenobia that I have detailed emanate from a man who is on the verge of infatuation, if not already over the edge. Fear of his own erotic desire prompts him to retreat into a rigid, phobic position: "for I should not, under any circumstances, have fallen in love with Zenobia" (p. 48).[8] Coverdale is hoist with his own petard: he turns away from an extraordinary woman, who could have enriched his lonely life immeasurably, and retreats, instead, to the reclusion of a voyeur and to affection for an asexual and unresponsive Priscilla, who Crews (1996) correctly judges is "a safer object of desire" (p. 201).[9] Given their many compatibilities of sensibility and intellect, an assertive Coverdale might have won over Zenobia's attention, which early on was fixed on Hollingsworth; but that would have made for a very different romance, if one at all.

Zenobia and Hollingsworth

The reader need not rely on Coverdale's observations of Zenobia's growing attachment to Hollingsworth, as Zenobia speaks volubly of it herself. She eagerly anticipates Hollingsworth's arrival at Blithedale as she had heard him lecture and was taken by him, not so much by what he said, which she does not comment on, but by his compelling manner: "What a voice he has! And what a man he is! Yet not so much an intellectual man, I should say, as a great heart; at least, he moved me more deeply than I think myself capable of being moved, except by the stroke of a true, strong heart next to my own" (p. 21). This is powerful sentiment: the prospect of a true heart stroking next to hers, as we shall see, engages Zenobia's profound emotional need. Although she is scornful of his devoting his "glorious powers" (p. 21) to the reformation of criminals [10], her heart overtakes her intellect and she will soon offer financial support for his project. There is also significant disparity in their interests and pursuits. Hollingsworth's magnetism lies outside the intellect; he is a blacksmith who expresses antipathy toward literary and other intellectual matters. Zenobia can be playfully sarcastic with Coverdale but maintains a solemnity toward Hollingsworth: "I cannot conceive of being so continually…within the sphere of a strong and noble nature, without being strengthened and ennobled by its influence!" (p. 68). The combination of manly strength and a tender heart is potent lure for Zenobia; as Coverdale attests there was "a tenderness in his voice, eyes, mouth, in his gesture, and in every indescribable manifestation, which few men could resist and no woman" (p. 28).

No incompatibility, however, is more problematic than that of Zenobia's deeply held convictions about the rights of women set against Hollingsworth's male chauvinism. Zenobia's feminist spirit is compromised by an idealization of Hollingsworth and a potent fear of his rejection. This is evident from the first night at Blithedale when Hollingsworth disapproves of her reception of Priscilla. Coverdale observes: "I think he positively frowned at Zenobia…he now looked stern and reproachful; and it was with that inauspicious meaning in his glance, that Hollingsworth first met Zenobia's eyes, and began his influence upon her life" (pp. 28–29).[11] Zenobia loses her self-possession and is "mortified and confused" (p. 29) as she responds to his stern look "almost humbly" (p. 29), "You do not quite do me justice, Mr. Hollingsworth" (p. 29). Her sensitivity to his reproof is again manifest at Eliot's Pulpit when her critique that "He [Man] is never content, unless he can degrade himself by stooping towards what he loves" (p. 122) is countered by what Coverdale calls the "masculine egotism" (p. 123) of Hollingsworth's retort: "The heart of true womanhood knows where its own sphere is, and never seeks to stray beyond it!" (p. 123). Rather than being indignant, Zenobia is again "humbled" (p. 123) and capitulates, "Well; be it so…I, at least, have deep cause to think you right. Let man be but manly and godlike, and woman is only too ready to become to him what you say!" (p. 124). Zenobia voices an unhappy awareness of a vulnerability which compels her to cede her convictions to Hollingsworth, with his "manly and godlike" qualities, rather than contradict him and risk his rejection. This vulnerability represents a psychological fault-line which will give way under the weight of Hollingsworth's ultimate rejection.

Zenobia is taken to task by critics for having attached herself to Hollingsworth as yet another mistake in her choice of men. Ullén (2004) judges that "she has willingly wasted her figurative fortune which is passionate love—on the wrong man, not once, but twice" (p. 236). I think that this is not an entirely fair assessment. There was much that was appealing about Hollingsworth that was in distinct contrast to the heartless Westervelt. Despite his burly appearance, he was a man "with such a soft place in his heart" (Hawthorne, 1962, Vol. 3, p. 42) and was capable, in Coverdale's experience, of a tenderness which was "the reflection of God's own love" (p. 43). He was a religious man and, however misguided Zenobia may have thought the project, he was, after all, a zealous advocate for the reform of an unprivileged segment of society. Coverdale concurs with Zenobia's estimation of him as a uniquely compelling speaker and he employs superlatives regarding his orations at Eliot's Pulpit: "No other speech of man has ever moved me like some of those discourses" (p. 119). Even after Hollingsworth dismisses her, Zenobia recalls the best of their times together: "But, we have come, many times before, to this grey rock, and we have talked very softly, among the whisperings of the birch-trees. They were pleasant hours!" (p. 216). While Coverdale's narrative, perhaps tellingly, does not record any generous sentiment offered by Hollingsworth toward Zenobia, the reader can imagine that a tender interchange provoked the gesture of avowal that Coverdale witnessed: "I plainly saw Zenobia take the hand of Hollingsworth in both her own, press it to her bosom, and let it fall again!" (p. 124). Unlike Coverdale, Zenobia was unable to resist Hollingsworth who succeeds in enlisting her in his cause "by addressing whatever is best and noblest in her" (p. 134). Perhaps, he sweetened the appeal by offering an appropriately gendered version of what he had proclaimed to Coverdale: "there is not the man in this wide world, whom I can love as I could love you" (p. 133). In refusing to join his project, Coverdale finds out sooner than Zenobia that an all-devouring egotism had overtaken and dehumanized Hollingsworth: "But, by-and-by, you missed the tenderness of yesterday, and grew conscious that Hollingsworth had a closer friend than every you could be. And this friend was the cold, spectral monster...his philanthropic theory!" (p. 55). Zenobia continues, almost to the end, to defend him and his singular project to Coverdale: "But a great man...attains his normal condition only through the inspiration of one great idea" (p. 166). Undoubtedly, with her heart engaged, Zenobia feared alienating him; unconscious denial inhibited her awareness of the baleful change in his personality. With his rejection of her after the loss of her fortune, the denial breaks down suddenly and painfully: "The utmost that can be said in your behalf—and because I would not be wholly despicable in my own eyes, but would fain excuse my wasted feelings, nor own it was wholly a delusion, therefore I say it – is, that a great and rich heart has been ruined in your breast" (p. 219).

The combination of manly strength and a woman's tender heart drives Zenobia's deep emotional attachment to Hollingsworth, often contrary to the voice of intellect and the inclinations of her otherwise commanding personality. In her idealization of him, in her fear to confront him or provoke his reproach, and in her denial of the erosion of his generous humanity, Zenobia is a woman under the sway of potent unconscious forces, the nature of which can be understood as having arisen from the traumatic circumstances of her childhood.

Fauntleroy

Coverdale's interview with Old Moodie, whose reticent tongue he purposefully loosens with drink, yields invaluable information for a psychoanalytic inquiry. Old Moodie, designated by Coverdale as Fauntleroy, of prodigious wealth earlier in his life, was a man of "no innate worth" (p. 183) whose being "crystallized itself into an external splendor" (p. 182) and had "no other life than upon this gaudy surface" (p. 182). However, his wife, Zenobia's mother, is characterized as "a lovely woman, whose nature was deeper than his own" (p. 182). Fauntleroy did not "keep this noble creature in his heart" (p. 182); rather he wore "her beauty for the most brilliant ornament of his outward state" (p. 182). Here is a foreshadowing of Zenobia's fate: like her mother, she is a lovely woman, of deep and noble nature, who longs for a man to take her into his heart but, instead, is used as an object of self-aggrandizement. Fauntleroy treats his child as he does his wife in that he took his "beautiful daughter from the beneficent hand of God with no just sense of her immortal value, but as a man already rich in gems, would receive another jewel. If he loved her, it was because she shone" (p. 182). A husband with this character will erode his wife's morale; however, a father like this can undermine his child's developing sense of self-worth. Zenobia was not given unconditional acceptance by her father; instead, the love that she received, if any, was contingent on gratifying his need to feel exalted through her. Old Moodie, in the encounter with Zenobia that he initiates, and whom he has not seen in years, demonstrates the persistence of this dynamic. After she departs, he exclaims, "Ah, but in Zenobia, I live again!...Let the world admire her, and be dazzled by her, the brilliant child of my prosperity! It is Fauntleroy that still shines through her!" (p. 192). Zenobia's remonstrance of Hollingsworth can to be understood as a response to what is a repetition of the egotistical cast of her father's relationship to her: "And you took me, too, into your plan, as long as there was hope of my being available, and now fling me aside again, a broken tool!" (p. 218).

Fauntleroy exhausts his fortune, commits a crime, and flees, thereby abandoning his family without material support. Zenobia's mother's fate is telescoped in the stark cadence of this line: "He fled; his wife perished by the necessity of her innate nobleness, in its alliance with a being so ignoble" (p. 183). The reader does not learn how Zenobia's mother "perished," but suicide is not out of the question. Be that as it may, the conflict between her noble nature and the ignominy she was stained with through Fauntleroy is a fatal one, as the same conflict proves to be for Zenobia years later. Zenobia's identification with her mother proves to be central to her destiny and is an example of Nancy Chodorow's (1978) assertion that a daughter "learns what it is to be womanlike in the context of this personal identification with her mother" (p. 175).

With her mother's death, Zenobia is bereft of her only secure source of love and is also shadowed by her father's shame: "betwixt her mother's death, and her father's ignominy, his daughter was left worse than orphaned" (p. 183). The death of a parent at an early age always has a momentous impact on a child's development and Zenobia is no exception. Without the compensatory love of the surviving parent or parent-surrogate, and without assistance in grieving and mourning, a child is apt to internalizes the loss as evidence of worthlessness. Such was Zenobia's circumstance with respect to the departed Fauntleroy: she was indeed a "forsaken child" (p. 189). Zenobia's life-story bears the mark of early loss and abandonment: a psyche burdened by a reservoir of grief and driven by longings for love and affection to compensate for those which were lost. Within this psychological matrix, rejection by a loved object evokes painful and often overpowering feelings associated with early parental loss. Regarding the aspects of her relationship to Hollingsworth that are manifestly under the influence of irrational forces, I suggest that Zenobia had unconsciously fastened on Hollingsworth, despite many obvious incompatibilities, for his unique melding of maternal and paternal qualities. Commenting on Hollingsworth's tenderness, Coverdale states: "But there was something of the woman molded into the great, stalwart frame of Hollingsworth" (p. 42). From the depths of the haunted mind, where still reside the wishes of a "forsaken child," Zenobia is drawn to Hollingsworth as "the one true heart to encourage and direct me, [that] might have made me all that a woman can be!" (p. 218). In her sensitivity to Hollingsworth's intolerance for dissent and the "stern and reproachful" (p. 28) glances that express it, Zenobia relives the instability of her father's love on which her sense of worth as a female child was, in significant measure, contingent. Hollingsworth's abrupt rejection re-evokes childhood feelings of abandonment and defectiveness: "It was my fault, all along, and none of his...What had I to offer him? A miserable, bruised and battered heart, spoilt long before he met me!" (p. 225).

As a child, Zenobia is saved from desolation by being taken in by her father's wealthy brother who provided the means to promote her "native graces" (p. 189), and consequently, "[i]n her triumphant progress toward womanhood, she was adorned with every variety of feminine accomplishment" (p. 189). Under this more fortunate circumstance, Zenobia was able to develop innate capacities and became the distinguished woman we see at Blithedale.[12] Her uncle dies, also when she is a child; his wealth will subsequently purchase various opportunities for her but not protection. The narrator insightfully notes: "she lacked a mother's care;" consequently, "With no adequate control on hand... her character was left to shape itself" (p. 189). Given her nature, which was "warm and generous," but also "[p]assionate, self-willed, and imperious," (p. 189) she needed, the narrator judiciously contends, a mother's guidance to help her through the instinctual perils which attend the passage from childhood into womanhood.[13] At Blithedale, Zenobia is aware that Priscilla is entering the same perilous phase of development and offers herself to her as a maternal figure, one that she lacked in adolescence: "you are getting to be so very pretty that you absolutely need a duenna; as I am older than you, and have had my own little experience of life, and think myself exceedingly sage, I intend to fill the place of a maiden-aunt" (p. 77).

Zenobia and Westervelt

In the absence of a mother's guidance, a young woman may go terribly astray in her love life. This is true for Zenobia as it is for Hester in *The Scarlet Letter* and Miriam in *The Marble Faun*. Zenobia's efflorescence into womanhood must have been stunning; the exotic flower that she wore daily at Blithedale was, she nostalgically admits, the "one relic of my more brilliant, my happier days!" (p. 45). Fate and instinct conspired against Zenobia to shorten those days: "There were whispers of an attachment, and even a secret marriage, with a fascinating and accomplished, but unprincipled young man" (p. 189). Undoubtedly, this man was the urbane, suave, educated, and unscrupulous Westervelt. Tellingly, Coverdale remarks that he was "as handsome a man as ever I beheld" (p. 91) and undoubtedly Zenobia refers this allure when she recalls to Coverdale, "[a]nd beauty, in a man, has been of little account with me, since my earliest girlhood, when, for once, it turned my head" (p. 227). Zenobia's liaison with Westervelt, like young Hester's marriage to Chillingworth in *The Scarlet Letter* took place "in the time when her heart knew no better"(Hawthorne, 1962, Vol. 1, p. 176). For Zenobia, the promptings of *Eros* held sway; a young woman of that time and place needed make such a mistake but "for once" to set her life on a path to misery from which there was no way back. Thus, both Zenobia and her mother were drawn to men who "glittered in the eyes of the world" (p. 182) but were eventually found to be emotionally hollow and cruelly insensitive. I believe that Coverdale, in his speculation as to what befell Zenobia in relation to Westervelt, although he is wide of the mark about other things, is deadly accurate about this: "How many a woman's evil fate has yoked her with a man like this! ...[who is] incomplete, on the emotional side, with hardly any sensibilities except for what pertain to us as animals...when a woman wrecks herself on such a being, she ultimately finds that the real womanhood, within her, has no corresponding part in him. Her deepest voice lacks a response; the deeper her cry, the more dead the silence....But the wretchedness, on her side, and the moral deterioration attendant on a false and shallow life, without strength enough to keep itself sweet, are amongst the most pitiable wrongs that mortals suffer" (p. 103). Zenobia would seem to confirm this speculation when she reveals a woman's suffering in the Legend of "The Silvery

Veil:" beneath the veil of her prodigiously beautiful appearance, her manifold capacities and material splendor, Zenobia feels herself, like The Veiled Lady, to be "a sad and lonely prisoner, in a bondage which is worse to me than death" (pp. 112–113).[14]

The reader is never told the exact nature of Zenobia's link to Westervelt, nor, I believe, is it essential to know. Ullén (2004) argues convincingly that they had been and are still married, and that this, Zenobia's secret, constitutes the indissoluble bond to him (p. 236). This conjecture does make sense of several elusive aspects of the narrative. Westervelt insinuates to Coverdale that he has been among Zenobia's "private friends" (p. 92): "Perhaps I might put forth a claim, on your own grounds, to call the lady by a name so appropriate to her splendid qualities" (p. 93). The claim, if consonant with Ullén's hypothesis, is that he is her husband. Be that as it may, Zenobia's interchange with Westervelt in the forest that Coverdale witnessed at a distance, leads him to conclude that her scorn and anger are "the result of an intimate love — on Zenobia's part, at least —in days gone by, but which prolonged itself into as intimate a hatred, for all futurity" (p. 102). At Zenobia's funeral, Westervelt adds further evidence that supports Coverdale's speculation when he exclaims: "Love had failed her, you say! Had it never failed her before?" (p. 240).[15]

Having experienced the "pressure of exceptional misfortune" (p. 121) involved in love that failed with Westervelt, but perhaps still bound to him legally, Zenobia has good reason to expostulate against the constraints that marriage imposes on a woman's freedom. She concludes that a woman can never be happy "after discovering that fate has assigned her but one single event, which she must contrive to make the substance of her whole life" (p. 60). In her private life, Zenobia resists this limitation and frees herself to live a life separate from Westervelt.[16] In the more progressive European milieu, literary women such as George Sand, Mme. de Stael, and George Eliot liberated themselves from institutional marriage. In America in the 1840's, such a separation for a woman was a serious breach of societal rules. Undoubtedly the strength of Zenobia's personality and, above all, the power she could command through her wealth, allowed her to elude society's disapprobation: "the world never criticized her so harshly as it does most woman who transcend its rules. It almost yielded its assent, when it beheld her stepping out of the common path, and asserting the more extensive privileges of her sex, both theoretically and by her practice. The sphere of ordinary womanhood was felt to be narrower than her development required" (p. 190). Undoubtedly, Zenobia was motivated, in part, to reside at Blithedale because it afforded her the opportunity to help fashion a community that could allow women to be on a more equal footing with men, one that was, in Coverdale's estimation, "widely different from that of conventional society" (p. 72). Regarding intimate relations, the Blithedale community "seemed to authorize any individual, of either sex, to fall in love with any other, regardless of what would elsewhere be judged suitable and prudent" (p. 72).

In being deprived of her wealth, Zenobia loses the ability to purchase social privilege and latitude. As it turns out, her fortune was founded solely on her father's whim; without it she becomes, in more ways than one, a fallen woman. Although she was noble in character and queenly in demeanor, there was no status in republican society afforded to her as dispossessed "royalty." In this way, she shares Hepzibah Pyncheon's dilemma in *The House of the Seven Gables* who finds herself "at the instant of time when the patrician lady is to be transformed into the plebian woman" (Hawthorne, 1962, Vol. 2, p. 38). The unhappy truth, for both women, is that "In this republican country, amid the fluctuating waves of our social life, somebody is always at the drowning-point. The tragedy is enacted with as continual a repetition as that of a popular drama on a holiday; and, nevertheless, is felt as deeply, perhaps, as when a hereditary noble sinks below his order. More deeply; since, with us, rank is the grosser substance of wealth and a splendid establishment, and has no spiritual existence after the death of these, but dies hopelessly along with them" (Hawthorne, 1962, Vol. 2, p. 38). As it relates to the consequences of her abrupt descent from prosperity to poverty, this passage provides a societal context of Zenobia's suicide.

At her funeral, Westervelt voices to Coverdale the fantasy that Zenobia would fall back into his control and that he could use her, as he did Priscilla, as an object of commerce: "She is now beyond my reach. Had she lived, and hearkened to my counsels, we might have served each other well" (p. 241). As was true of her mother, Zenobia is "hopelessly entangled" (p. 225) with a villain proved to be "indissoluble, except by death" (p. 240).

Zenobia and Priscilla

With Priscilla's appearance at Blithedale, as if *ex nihilo,* Zenobia encounters her "evil fate" (p. 220). In a penetrating essay, Angela Mills (2003) considers Zenobia and Priscilla's sisterhood, "literal and figurative...to be at the heart of the tale" (p. 98). Priscilla, whose mother also died when she was a child, was raised in social deprivation by Old Moodie. As a symptom of her desolation, Priscilla "devoutly loved" (Hawthorne, 1962, Vol. 3, p. 186), in a way that was "almost like worship," (p. 186)her older sister whom she had never met, but whose beauty and wealth Old Moodie has vaunted to her. Priscilla's removal to Blithedale was arranged by Old Moodie in order for her to find refuge there under Zenobia's protection from Westervelt, to whom she was enthralled as the celebrated Veiled Lady. Undoubtedly following Old Moodie's instructions, when she arrives at Blithedale, Priscilla withholds her identity as Zenobia's sister.[17] This proves to be a fatal secret. For all her purported love for her sister, Priscilla's relationship with Zenobia at Blithedale is essentially dishonest. Old Moodie has set up what Ullén rightly considers a "rather cruel experiment" (p. 217) which seeks to determine if Zenobia will treat Priscilla as she would a sister without knowing their true relation. This is yet another iteration of the scheme that Old Moodie created long before that pitted one sister against the other: rather than use the wealth he inherited from his brother to benefit both children, he gives access to all the fortune, for a time, to Zenobia, and keeps himself and Priscilla in poverty. As part of sending Priscilla to Blithedale, he sets up this test for Zenobia which, by its nature, she is doomed to fail, and consequently, then punishes her by transferring his entire wealth to Priscilla. Mills accurately assesses that their father "masterminded conditions that will help direct the course of his daughters' relationship" (p. 109). Old Moodie takes pleasure in the role of a *deus absconditus*.[18]

Priscilla affixes herself to the person of her sister in a manner bizarre enough to lead Zenobia to conjecture that she is deranged. Her plea to Hollingsworth is that Zenobia, who has never seen her before, "will shelter me...and let me be always near her!" (p. 29). In addition, the dazed girl is fearful, inarticulate, and physically wasted. In not being hampered by Coverdale's penchant to poeticize Priscilla, Zenobia sees her for what she is: a pathetic and malnourished young woman who has been the victim of male domination. Zenobia exclaims: "Poor thing! She has been stifled with the heat of a salamander-stove, in a small, close room, and has drunk coffee, and fed upon dough-nuts, raisins, candy, and all such trash until she is scarcely half-alive" (p. 34). Zenobia's instincts prove correct: in his interview with Old Moodie, Coverdale discovers that Priscilla had indeed grown up confined in an overcrowded chamber. She had rarely been beyond its walls and when she did venture out, she was the object of mockery by neighbors because of her oddity. In the absence of exercise, her muscles were weak and poor coordinated; when first at Blithedale she was unable to run without falling. Although a late adolescent in age, she was not yet pubescent, a symptom of retarded sexual development due to chronic malnutrition. Westervelt, who had paid visits to Priscilla in her dwelling, had visible evidence on which to base his judgment that her nervous fragility was the product of "unwholesome food, bad air, lack of out-door exercise, and neglect of bathing" (p. 95). Nina Baym (1968) is in accord that Priscilla "is simply a victim, her physical and mental disabilities directly caused by her exploited life" (p. 262). Priscilla's only talent, apart from clairvoyance, was sewing, which Old Moodie put to work as a means to raise money; the bags she fashioned, like herself, were without volume. There is nothing to suggest that she received an education. Thus, Priscilla's upbringing under Old Moodie was severely impoverished, and unnecessarily so; one can imagine what she endured under the control of the miscreant, Westervelt, with whom she was "enthralled in an intolerable bondage, from which she must either free herself or perish" (p. 190).[19]

The young woman's emotional life was markedly constricted. Priscilla was capable of love, but only in the form of blind devotion and to only one person. She attempts to exclude painful memories from awareness, although they return to haunt her in the form of dissociative experiences. Old Moodie, however, remembers what Priscilla will not: "if she were to see this old face of mine, the child would remember some very sad times, which we have spent together. Some very sad times indeed!" (p. 85). As a consequence of the neglect and abuse she suffered, her sense of having a self that can initiate choice and action is virtually non-existent: she avows "I am blown about like a leaf…I never have any free-will" (p. 171). And a leaf does not think: an impartial reader who examines everything that Priscilla says over the course of the narrative will not find a single thoughtful utterance. This vacancy within the structure of the self, however, creates the conditions that facilitate her abilities as a medium.[20]

There is not sufficient emphasis in the critical literature that, after their initial encounter, Zenobia treats Priscilla with kindness and protective solicitude. Under her care, and Hollingsworth's, Priscilla matures physically and her fearful and withdrawn demeanor becomes cheerful and spirited. Zenobia's natural generosity extends itself to her, even without the knowledge that Priscilla is her sibling: "I neither know nor care what it is in me that so attaches her. But she loves me, and I will not fail her" (p. 104). It is not until Zenobia has evidence Priscilla is her rival that she is incited to hostility toward her. Vexed by Priscilla's peculiar attachment to her the first night at Blithedale, Zenobia comments to Coverdale: "However, I am positively not an ill-natured person, unless when very grievously provoked" (p. 34). Hollingsworth, in recklessly soliciting the affections of both, has, as Coverdale astutely perceives, set up a dangerous rivalry: "for a girl like Priscilla, and a woman like Zenobia, to jostle one another in their love of a man like Hollingsworth, was likely to be no child's play" (p. 72). Although for very different reasons, both Old Moodie and Hollingsworth create the conditions for a destructive contest between the two. That both Zenobia and Priscilla are exploited by Old Moodie, Westervelt and Hollingsworth is one aspect of the romance's "fearful symmetry."

The rivalry is brought to a crisis that Coverdale predicted, when Westervelt appears at Blithedale and seeks an interview with Zenobia. Although Coverdale cannot clearly discern the content of their interchange, the reader discovers its essentials in Zenobia's Legend, "The Silvery Veil." What Coverdale does hear is Zenobia's tormented exclamation regarding Westervelt: "With what kind of being am I linked!…if my Creator cares aught for my soul, let him release me from this miserable bond!…it will strangle me at last!" (p. 104).

The Legend of "The Silvery Veil"

The vigilant Coverdale observes that, "Since her interview with Westervelt, Zenobia's continual inequalities of temper had been rather difficult for her friends to bear" (pp. 119–120). Indeed, her meeting with Westervelt, the romance's *peripeteia*, precipitates a crisis that sets in motion the trajectory to her death.[21] The anxieties related to the peril she now feels, and the moral conflicts that had been incited by it, find expression in the Legend of "The Silvery Veil," which she narrates to the Blithedale community the next evening. In this spontaneous dramatic monologue, her oratorical *magnum opus,* Zenobia's transforms urgent psychic conflicts into artistic representation. *Pari passu*, this gives the reader a glimpse into the psychological dynamics of Hawthorne's creative process.[22]

The first part of the Legend presents an allegory of Zenobia's quest for love. Baym (1968) observes that "In this story, Zenobia is actually assimilating the Veiled Lady into herself" (p. 262). Indeed, the celebrated woman in the Legend stands for Zenobia, whose striking public persona invites speculation, especially from men, about her secret life. At the beginning of the novel, Coverdale suggests this interpretation when he asserts that "Zenobia… is merely her public name; a sort of mask in which she comes before the world, retaining all the privileges of privacy—a contrivance, in short, like the white drapery of the Veiled Lady, only a little more transparent" (p. 8). The Legend captures Zenobia's unhappy fate as a woman whose secret is more important for others to know than the qualities that characterize the "immortal value" of her being. When The Veiled Lady enters the private drawing-room, "She was in quest of something!" (p. 112). Her ensuing drama with Theodore expresses a longing for a man whose love encompasses her as a generously loving woman who, like everyone, has a secret. Her question to Theodore becomes a lament: "Hast not thy heart recognized me?" (p. 113). The answer is "no," as it had been for Zenobia in relation to her father and Westervelt and, as she will soon discover, to Hollingsworth. As Mitchell (1998) points out, the interchange with the Legend's seeker, Theodore, reflects the conversation that she had with Coverdale while he was convalescing (p. 182). The Veiled Lady's question to Theodore, "What wouldst thou with me?" (p. 112) finds its parallel in Zenobia's question to Coverdale upon becoming aware that he is intently observing her: "What are you seeking to discover in me?" (p. 47). Theodore's response, "Mysterious creature…I would know who and what you are!" (p. 112) mirrors Covedale's reply to Zenobia: "The mystery of your life… And you will never tell me" (p. 47). In spite of the many extraordinary qualities of her character that Coverdale has observed and recorded, his answer betokens more interest in what is hidden than what is manifest. Rather than allowing herself to be the object of scrutiny, Zenobia challenges him to participate with her in a mutual gaze: "She bent her head toward me, and let me look into her eyes" (pp. 47–48). Coverdale sees only a projection of his own fear: "I see nothing now … unless it be the face of a sprite, laughing at me from the bottom of a deep well" (p. 48). His eyes probe but his heart does not recognize what they see.[23] And like Theodore who is left quite alone after The Veiled Lady vanishes, with Zenobia's death, Coverdale's "retribution was to pine, forever and ever, for another sight of that dim, mournful face" (p. 114). The Veiled Lady departs bearing an "inexpressible sadness" (p. 113).

Under the pressure of immanent events, the second part of the Legend shifts from allegory to verisimilitude. In it, the narrator is warned by the Magician that her prospects for love and fortune are threatened by the maiden who "comes out of the realm of Mystery" (p. 115) and appeared in the Blithedale community's midst. The Magician insists that only way to thwart the threat is for her to throw the silvery veil over the maiden and then call for him. The maiden will thus be returned to his control; after this is accomplished, the Magician reassures her, "you are safe!" (p. 115). This is Zenobia's thinly-disguised account of the conversation the previous day which can now be reconstructed: Westervelt informed her that Priscilla is, in fact, The Veiled Lady who had been in his control and he wants her back. Westervelt informs Zenobia she is in imminent danger of losing both fortune and love to Priscilla. Undoubtedly by employing some form of extortion based on their prior relationship, he demands that Zenobia use her influence to deliver Priscilla to him in exchange for his removing the threat that she poses.[24] The Legend makes clear that Zenobia, despite the horror and disgust she holds toward Westervelt's proposal, has already decided to accede to it. At the end of the recitation, she throws the veil over Priscilla thereby signaling her intention, *in flagrante delicto*. The moral conflict that Zenobia experiences over this proposed action is represented in the look the narrator of the Legend reads in the maiden's eyes as she performs the act of betrayal: "the poor girl strove to raise it, and met her dear friend's eyes with one glance of mortal terror, and deep, deep reproach. It could not change her purpose" (p. 116). The power of the returned glance reasserts itself. The reproach the narrator sees is, of course, a projection of Zenobia's conscience: she knows Westervelt only too well and that returning Priscilla to him is morally wrong. In Freudian terms, and how barren they sound, the promptings of the id surmount the prohibitions of the superego. Zenobia articulates this conflict when she later admits to Priscilla, "You stood between me and an end that I desired. I wanted a clear path" (p. 220). Nor is the conspiracy with Westervelt, given the moral conflict that inheres in it, easy for her to execute: upon his leave-taking from Blithedale, Coverdale observes in Zenobia's eyes "a troubled and passionate flame, flickering and fitful" (p. 141). She senses an oncoming catastrophe and states to him, self-mockingly yet truthfully, that she needs a confidant with whom she can "share the bosom-secrets of a tragedy-queen" (p. 142) or a counsellor, be it "an angel or a madman," who could serve as "wild steersman when we voyage through Chaos!" (p. 142). Instead, she is utterly alone.

The reader needs to remember that Zenobia did not yet know that Priscilla was her half-sister. It is inconceivable that she would have returned her to Westervelt had she known this. Had she been aware of their true relation, she told Priscilla "some things, that have chanced, might have been spared you" (p. 220). Old Moodie's secret experiment becomes malignant for both daughters. In the end, Zenobia asks Priscilla for forgiveness: "It is over now. Do you forgive me?" (p. 220). Mills (2003) concludes, severely, that Zenobia failing her sister is "her greatest shame, her measure of self-defeat" (p. 100). Zenobia need not be reminded of this as her stern superego will not be placated and exacts its punishment; her action against Priscilla stains her for the brief remainder of her life. After Hollingsworth rejects her, she excoriates herself: "I am a woman—with every fault, it may be, that a woman ever had, weak, vain, unprincipled... passionate, too, and pursuing my foolish and unattainable ends, by indirect and cunning, though absurdly chosen means" (p. 217). That she had led another woman back to the domination of a man was a betrayal of principle; she judges herself as having been "false, moreover, to the whole circle of good, in my reckless truth to the little good I saw before me..." (pp. 217–218). This unsparing moral reckoning is a crucial part of Zenobia's stature as a tragic figure.

Zenobia made good on her part of the bargain, but Westervelt does not deliver on his. It is never clear how Westervelt convinced Zenobia he could neutralize the threat that Priscilla posed. Perhaps he had a viable scheme or, just as likely, he had none and was manipulating her to gain his end. He is, after all, a villain. In the end, the result is antithetical to what he promised. Ironically, the Magician's statement, "You are safe!" applies rather to Priscilla, not Zenobia. Old Moodie, who had all along kept himself informed as to Priscilla's status at Blithedale, must have learned of her abduction by Westervelt and Zenobia's part in it. Having contemplated something of the sort in the very recent past, he is now prompted to take definitive action against Zenobia by transferring his fortune entirely to Priscilla.[25]

Hollingsworth learns of Zenobia's reversal of fortune, rescues Priscilla from Westervelt at a Village-Hall and returns her to Blithedale. In the midst of all this action, which is out of Coverdale's sight and thus the reader's, it is likely that Zenobia's relationship to Westervelt, her long-held secret, has been made public and is a source of shame for her. Zenobia tells Coverdale that a woman in her position "would be apt to blush, too, under the eyes that knew her secret; her heart might throb uncomfortably" (p. 225). It would seem that Hollingsworth takes the opportunity the revelation of this secret affords him to end his relationship with Zenobia. It is unlikely that his rejection of Zenobia is prompted by her part in turning Priscilla over to Westervelt, as some critics have suggested, since he also conspired in that plot.[26] Hollingsworth's "dark, self-delusive egotism" (p. 79) prevents him from being aware that the transformation of his hitherto fraternal feelings into "love" toward Priscilla coincides precisely with her becoming a wealthy woman. With this change in Hollingsworth's affections, so clearly following the direction of who has the money, Zenobia forcefully denounces his character. Her idealization of him finally breaks down: "I see it now! I am awake, disenchanted, disenthralled! Self, self, self!" (p. 218). However, the damage has been done. Mills (2003) perceptively concludes that Hollingsworth's choice of Priscilla "is a crushing rebuke to Zenobia...Not only is the materialistic nature of Hollingsworth's interest in the women exposed in his pursuit of cash, but he signals that, for him, the sisters are entirely interchangeable, part of the general traffic in women. Zenobia's education, intelligence, refinement and beauty rate little in Hollingsworth's calculation" (p. 108).

Zenobia's Suicide

In the last days of her life, Zenobia is confronted with revelations and reversals that press upon her with relentless force. She has learned that the decrepit man she had recently met within his squalid chamber is her father and that he has kept himself hidden from her for years. All along, the fortune she thought was hers and the status it afforded her in society was in his control; he has just dispossessed her of both. The insubstantial Priscilla is revealed as her half-sister, and has claimed victory over her in love and fortune, and without a backward glance. In being drawn into a plot with Westervelt, she betrayed her principles, and is burdened with self-reproach and shame; the plot has failed and she is still not free of the miscreant. As the coup de grâce, Hollingsworth, the man whose great heart she had sought, has abandoned her; the blow has lighted "on a woman's heart, over which she wears no breastplate" (p. 224).[27]

The unconscious also has its say in Zenobia's fate. Reduced to the prospect of poverty and in desolation, Zenobia has again been "left worse than orphaned" (p. 183). Under these conditions, which recreate the traumata of her childhood, the vaults of the haunted mind are flung open and she is flooded with painful feelings that arise from that troubled era. Coverdale's description of Zenobia during the terrible moments at Eliot's Pulpit bears repetition: "...she began slowly to sink down. It was as if a great, invisible, irresistible weight were pressing her to the earth. Settling upon her knees, she leaned her forehead against the rock, and sobbed convulsively; dry sobs, they seemed to be, such as have nothing to do with tears" (p. 221). By the time she becomes aware that Coverdale has been observing her and she collects herself, the decision to end her life has already been made; everything in her ensuing interchange with Coverdale points to that resolve.

What Zenobia experienced during that dark interval remains hidden within the sanctity of her human heart. I offer the following construction as an attempt to further an understanding of her and her subsequent action. As she is bent against the rock, she relives her past as a "forsaken child" (p. 189). She experiences, in overwhelming waves, the inchoate and ineffable anguish associated with her mother's death. As these memories are evoked, I imagine what ensues in Zenobia's mind by recalling lines from William Wordsworth's *Tintern Abbey*:

> Oh! then,
> If solitude, or fear, or pain, or grief,
> Should be thy portion, with what healing thoughts
> Of tender joy wilt thou remember me,
> And these my exhortations!

Through the work of the unconscious, Zenobia is drawn together with her mother as "the one true heart to encourage and direct me" (p. 218). In *Mourning and Melancholia*, Freud elucidates the mechanism of identification with the lost object. This identification now guides her action: Zenobia's noble character, of necessity, repels the ignominy in which she finds herself; as did her mother, she must perish in order to be released from it. In sharing her mother's end, she communes with a "woman's doom" (p. 223) and accepts it with a nobility of sentiment that arouses pathos and awe: "I have deserved it like a woman; so let there be no pity, as on my part, there shall be no complaint" (pp. 223–224). That choosing death has finally made her "all that a woman can be" (p. 218) is the essence of her tragic destiny.

Zenobia may succumb to fate without complaint, but not without defiance. The indictment she expresses to Coverdale is sweeping: "the whole universe, her own sex and yours, and Providence, or Destiny, to boot, make common cause against the woman who swerves one hair's breadth out of the beaten track" (p. 224). With these forces arrayed against her, Zenobia's struggle must end in defeat. Earlier she promises: "If I live another year, I will lift up my own voice, in behalf of woman's wider liberty" (p. 120). However, she had presciently warned that "The mistrust and disapproval of the vast bulk of society throttles us, as with two gigantic hands at our throats!" (p. 120). Her voice was silenced, but its message was inscribed for all time in *The Blithedale Romance.*

Zenobia not only reckons with society's strictures, but also with the momentous consequences of having deviated from them: "Yes, and add, (for I may as well own it, now) that, with that one hair's breadth, she goes all astray, and never sees the world in its true aspect, afterwards" (p. 224). In swerving outside of the boundaries set by society, she is removed from the circle of sympathy with it, and is thereby left "all astray." This is also Hester's dilemma in *The Scarlet Letter.* Zenobia's acceptance of her moral frailty and the painful limits of a struggle to oppose society constitute an *anagnorisis* in the tradition of Greek tragedy.[28] F.O. Matthiessen (1941) finds Zenobia one of Hawthorne's protagonists who "finally face their evil and know it deserving of the sternest justice, and thus participate in the purgatorial movement, the movement towards regeneration" (p. 350). In a beautiful appreciation of her character, he concludes that "there is no release for Zenobia save in death. Yet in such a figure...Hawthorne was most able to affirm the warmth and strength of the heart, and so to create a sense not merely of life's inexorability and sordidness, but of its possibilities of beauty and grandeur" (p. 155).

In a miracle of understatement, Hawthorne refers to Zenobia in the Preface as "the high-spirited Woman, bruising herself against the narrow limits of her sex" (Vol. 3, p. 2).[29] The bruise proved fatal. George Eliot (1852), in her magisterial review of the novel shortly after its publication, expresses affront at the fate the author assigns to Zenobia: "Zenobia is the only one of the group worthy to be the Trustee of Human Right, and the Representative of Human Destiny; and she, at least should have come out of her struggles in regal triumph" (p.66).[30] Hawthorne indeed provokes the reader's moral outrage that Zenobia ends in suicide. Eliot directs her anger at this outcome onto the author; Hawthorne, I believe, would rather have us turn it inward so that we examine the ways we make "common cause against" the womanhood represented so magnificently in Zenobia. The "bright hopes" (p. 227) for societal reform at Blithedale were "indeed, a foolish dream" (p. 227); Hawthorne has not deviated from the conclusion he reached in relation to the failed attempts at radical reform detailed in "Earth's Holocaust" (1844): "Purify that inner sphere; and the many shapes of evil that haunt the outward, and which now seems almost our only realities, will turn to shadowy phantoms, and vanish of their own accord" (Hawthorne, 1974, Vol. 10, 404). Richard H. Millington (1992) astutely assesses Hawthorne's moral intent in what he characterizes as *The Blithedale Romance*'s regenerative hostility: "He sets out, in his own chastened version of reform, to renovate his community of readers from the inside out" (p. 176).

Aftermath

One of the purposes of tragedy is to inform the moral lives of those who witness it. Zenobia, too often an object of projected fantasy, never found an affirmative answer to her searching question: "Hast thou not recognized me?" That she must wait to find recognition in death accords with the wisdom expressed in *The House of the Seven Gables*: "Death is so genuine a fact that it excludes falsehood, or betrays its emptiness; it is a touch-stone that proves the gold, and dishonors the baser metal" (Hawthorne, 1962, Vol. 2, p. 310). Death, the immitigable instructor in all Hawthorne's romances, reveals Zenobia's inestimable value.

At Zenobia's funeral, Old Moodie appears "in deep mourning, his face mostly concealed with a handkerchief" (Hawthorne, 1962, Vol. 3, p. 239). Tellingly, as her father, he takes his place in the procession "nearest the dead" (p. 239). What the narrator says of Matthew Maule vis à vis Alice Pyncheon in *The House of the Seven Gables* is equally true of Old Moodie's treatment of Zenobia: "He meant to humble Alice, not to kill her;–but, he had taken a woman's delicate soul into his rude gripe, to play with; — and she was dead!" (Vol. 2, p. 210). Zenobia's death may have imparted to him, finally, a "just sense of her immortal value" (p. 182). It was indeed Old Moodie's "fatality to behold whatever he touched dissolve" (p. 185).

Westervelt, devoid of emotion "except what pertains to us as animals" (p. 103), is moved only to cynical anger because Zenobia has extricated herself from him. Without a human heart, there can be no moral awakening. The reader replies with "amen" to Coverdale's exhortation to the higher powers: "Heaven deal with Westervelt according to his nature and deserts! —that is to say, annihilate him" (p. 241).

Undoubtedly, Coverdale never delivered Zenobia's imprecation to Hollingsworth: "Tell him he has murdered me! Tell him that I'll haunt him!" (p. 226) but Hollingsworth's superego carries out her charge. When Coverdale seeks him out years later, he is in a melancholic state "that seemed habitual" (p. 242); his physical and mental deterioration are evidence of the accuracy of Zenobia's surmise that he had severed their bond when he discovered that she could no longer fund his project. For that moral crime and its awful consequence, the stern tribunal of his conscience has returned a guilty verdict by which he is condemned to purgatorial suffering. He confesses to Coverdale, "Ever since we parted, I have been busy with a single murderer!" (p. 243). Upon first seeing him, Coverdale is filled with "bitter and revengeful emotion," but Hollingsworth's self-condemnation arouses him to leniency: "Then the tears gushed into my eyes, and I forgave him" (p. 243). Perhaps, in light of his penitent confession and the forgiveness it elicited, Hollingsworth will be afforded a redemptive path.

Coverdale had also fared poorly since Zenobia's death. The life he describes is characteristic of one burdened by persistent depression that has drained him of vitality and, as he admits, "rendered my own life all an emptiness" (p. 246). The confession that he would "rush at levelled bayonets," (p. 247) if he only had the energy to find a nearby battle, represents a fantasied enactment of a suicidal wish. His life, voided of meaning, amounts to: "Nothing, nothing, nothing!" (p. 245).

What ails Miles Coverdale? I would diagnose his paralyzed state as symptomatic of unresolved grief for the woman who captured his heart and whom he lost forever: Zenobia. Beneath his awareness, but nonetheless written throughout the interstices of his text, is abundant evidence of a deep attachment to her. Millicent Bell (1962) concludes, "One suspects, really, that he loved Zenobia" (p. 159).[31] Until he can experience what Zenobia meant to him, he is not able to grieve over what is unrecoverable in her death. All that is repressed in Coverdale's unconscious, finally pushes against the inertia of his depressed state and drives him to revisit Hollingsworth and Priscilla where the work of mourning can begin.

In order to justify this interpretation, I would need to explicate much more of Coverdale's psychology than is possible here, but one thing is certain: Coverdale hides from himself what was closest to his heart. Zenobia is the alpha and omega of his Blithedale experience. On his first day he remarks: "the presence of Zenobia caused our heroic enterprise to show like an illusion, a masquerade, a pastoral, a counterfeit Arcadia, in which we grown-up men and women were making a play-day of the years that were given us to live in. I tried to analyze this impression, but not with much success" (p. 21). If Coverdale had consulted his heart and not his head, he could have appreciated that within him was a burgeoning love for "truly a magnificent woman" (p. 44). He also should have taken more seriously the exalted sensation of her extraordinary "bloom, health and vigor" that "a man might well have fallen in love with her for their sake only" (p. 16). With Zenobia's death, Blithedale is depleted of meaning: "I left Blithedale within the week after Zenobia's death, and went back thither no more. The whole soil of our farm, for a long time afterwards, seemed but sodded earth over her grave" (p. 245).

Contrary to Coverdale's proclivity toward self-denigration, Zenobia did not underestimate him as a poet. In fact, she praised his "beautiful poetry"

(p. 14), and chided him periodically for not writing more faithfully, as she considers him one of the world's "true poets" (p. 14). Thus, the rhetorical question Zenobia poses regarding Hollingsworth was equally germane for Coverdale: "For will he never, in many an hour of darkness, need that proud, intellectual sympathy which he might have had from me?" (p. 225). Zenobia's intellectual vitality could have illuminated many hours of creative darkness for him. Without that kind of encouragement, his energies as a poet have failed him.[32] In the intervening years, he had "nobody but myself to care for" (p. 246) and thus nobody to care for him, a man who assuredly needed caring. Like Theodore in his encounter with the Legend's Veiled Lady, Coverdale had the possibility with Zenobia that "all the felicity of earth and of the future world shall by thine and mine together" (p. 113). Early in their relationship, when Zenobia asked "What do you seek to discover in me?" (p. 47), the truest answer, not available to him then, would have been simply, "love." Instead, and it was to his great misfortune, he turned away from a "pure and generous purpose" (p. 113) toward her in favor of "scornful scepticism and idle curiosity" (p. 113). That Zenobia includes this incident in her Legend, a clear reference to her relationship with him, suggests that, if he had recognized her, she could have been ready to receive and reciprocate his love. Instead, he is consigned to share Theodore's fate to "pine, forever and ever, for another sight of that dim, mournful face – which might have been his life-long, house-hold, fireside joy—to desire, and waste life in a feverish quest, and never meet it more!" (p. 114). Zenobia's and Coverdale's stars were misaligned. At the novel's end, Zenobia wistfully reflects on what could have been: "It is an endless pity…that I had not bethought myself of winning your heart, Mr. Coverdale, instead of Hollingsworth's. I think I should have succeeded…But there is a fate in these things" (pp. 226–227).

Coverdale's formidable defenses are breached when he again sees Hollingsworth and Priscilla. The "bitter and revengeful emotion" that erupts is hitherto repressed anger toward the man whose actions precipitated the loss of Zenobia to suicide; however, when he sees Hollingsworth's broken state, Coverdale feels both pity and forgiveness. And the tears that gush out of his eyes express the grief at her death that he had never permitted himself to experience. The gateway to his haunted mind has been opened.[33] His exquisite lines of homage reveal that he has come to recognize her: with Zenobia's death, he writes, Nature's highest purpose, "that of conscious, intellectual life, and sensibility had been baulked! While Zenobia lived, Nature was proud of her, and directed all eyes upon that radiant presence, as her fairest handiwork. Zenobia perished" (p. 244). This was, in short, Zenobia's story, and his. With his emotions and intellect congruent, Coverdale evokes the "irrepressible yearnings over the Blithedale reminiscences" (p. 246) and Zenobia's radiant presence at its center of them all; as an act of mourning that is conceived "by Zenobia's grave," he transforms her story into a "ballad," *The Blithedale Romance*. In accordance with her instruction, and in his unique way, he put his "soul's ache into it" (p. 224). Coverdale is united with Zenobia as his tragic muse.

Coverdale's concluding confession, about which rivers of ink have flowed, can be understood in light of the foregoing interpretation. "I—I myself—was in love—with—Priscilla!" (p. 247) is, indeed, "essential to the full understanding of my story" (p. 247). That a man such as Coverdale, who, like Zenobia, was of "diversified capacity" (p. 241), would seek love with a woman of such limited scope as Priscilla, bespeaks the profundity of his psychological compromise.[34] Coverdale reveals the truth about his psychology that has been manifest diversely throughout his emotional struggles at Blithedale: a fear of sexuality, a peremptory need to be the sole object of affection, a hypersensitivity to rejection, and a proclivity toward fantasy and obsession in the place of determined action. In a deep stratum of his psyche, lies a fragile sense of self. His having sought love with the "poor, pale flower," (p. 224) Priscilla, betrays these psychological vulnerabilities. It tells us who he was. With touching and profound self-awareness, as well as irony and pathos, Coverdale's confession offers the reader, in the subtlest manner, the full understanding of his story.

Notes

1. The characters' speculations as to Zenobia's motivation are in keeping with the attitudes toward suicide at the time. Albert Rhodes' 1876 study of suicide based on US federal census statistics suggests different motives between women and men: "Women appear to be more subject to moral influences such as disappointed love, betrayal, desertion, jealousy, domestic trouble and sentimental exaltation of every description." Men "are rather affected by trials of a material order, such as misery, business embarrassments, losses, ungratified ambition, the abuse of alcohol, the desire to escape from justice, and so on" (Kushner, 1985, p. 541). For an examination of suicide in Victorian England, including its representation in fiction, see Barbara Gates' (1988) *Victorian Suicide: Mad Crimes and Sad Histories.*
2. There is yet another murder suspect. Mary Suzanne Schriber (1982) contends that "Suicide over unrequited love is out of character for Zenobia" and suggest, instead, "that it seems plausible to suspect Hollingsworth of murdering her" (p. 74).
3. Regarding the subject of gender, Chodorow (1999) writes: "Whether racial-ethnic, international feminist, linguistic, performative, micropolitical, or based on the analysis of discourse, gender theories that do not consider individual and fantasy-related material cannot capture fully the meanings that gender has for the subject. They miss an important component of experienced gender meaning and gendered subjectivity" (p. 171). She makes the following methodologic recommendation: "we need to cross what might be called the horizontal view of cultural meaning–thick descriptions, multiplicity, polysemic webs of meaning, forest of symbols—with a vertical view, in which each individual's internal history is its own emotionally polysemic web of continually created unconscious and conscious personal meaning, animated by fantasies, projections, and introjections" (p. 173).
4. The Boston literary circle was undoubtedly familiar with the story of the Palmyrean Queen. Her life had been the subject of William Ware's popular epistolary romance, *Zenobia or The Fall of Palmyra*, published in 1837. After defying the Romans in battle, Zenobia was captured and, according

to many sources, transported to Rome where she was paraded through the populace in shackles. Harriet Hosmer, a friend of Hawthorne, captured the moment in her famous sculpture, "Zenobia in Chains" (1859). In suicide, the *Blithedale* Zenobia escapes her namesake's public humiliation.

5. Ryan Stuart Lowe (2017) comments, "if critics have been sensitive to Margaret Fuller's feminism as a possible source for Zenobia, they have often overlooked the influence of George Sand's reputation as a gender-bending author and a free lover" (pp. 68–69).
6. I believe that Gordon Beauchamp (2002) underestimates the seriousness of Zenobia's commitment to social reform expressed in her taking up residence at Blithedale when he opines, "Zenobia's true motive for coming to Blithedale is the quite un-feminist one of trying to catch a husband–Hollingsworth, to be exact" (p. 44).
7. Thomas R. Mitchell's *Hawthorne's Fuller Mystery* (1998) is a thoughtful consideration of the impact of Hawthorne's relationship with Margaret Fuller on his writings, including his rendering of Zenobia. The book is essentially a psychological study of Hawthorne, but does not articulate a psychological theory or set of theories upon which its conclusions are based. A writer's life inevitably finds its way into his or her work; the issue which Mitchell does not explore is how Hawthorne transforms his biography into literary art.
8. Zenobia complains to Coverdale that in Priscilla's effusive display of affection toward her, she is being offered "...a little more love than one can conveniently dispose of; –and that, let me say, Mr. Coverdale, is the most troublesome offense you can offer a woman" (p. 34). Ever sensitive to rebuff, Coverdale replies to Zenobia's comment as if she had issued an admonition specifically for him: "Thank you!...I don't mean to be guilty of it" (p. 34). Coverdale kept his word.
9. At no time did Priscilla show an interest in Coverdale. Each attempt he makes to engage her is deflected, discouraged or simply not responded to. Coverdale's attachment to her is nurtured entirely by fantasy.
10. Zenobia comments to Coverdale: "I should like Mr. Hollingsworth a great deal better, if the philanthropy had been left out" (p. 22).
11. Zenobia's destiny is decided in a glance, as it was for Donatello in *The Marble Faun*, when holding the Model over the precipice, his eyes met Miriam's.
12. Commenting on Zenobia's capacities, Coverdale states, "She was made (among a thousand other things that she might have been) for a stump-oratress" (p. 44).
13. Coverdale is consistent in his characterization of the child's need to have limits set by his mother. In another context he compares nature to "a strict but loving mother, who uses the rod upon her little boy for his naughtiness, and gives him a smile, a kiss and some pretty playthings, to console the urchin for her severity" (p. 62). Nothing is written about Zenobia's uncle's relationship with her. In any case, the narrator offers the following gendered assessment: "a man, however stern...can never sway and guide a female child" (p. 189).
14. Citing the same passage, Pfister (1991) makes the following observation about the Veiled Lady: "Although she most resembles Priscilla, one cannot help but hear the voice of Zenobia in her plea to Theodore" (p. 91).
15. In Zenobia's Legend, The Veiled Lady entreats Theodore, "in all maiden modesty, to bend forward, and impress a kiss, where my breath stirs the veil; and my virgin lips shall come forward to meet thy lips" (p. 113). Through The Veiled Lady, Zenobia is telling her own story which, as she intimates in

this sentence, has not been marked by sexual experience. Being married is not necessarily equivalent to being sexually experienced. There is reason to believe, in *The Scarlet Letter*, that Hester's marriage to Chillingworth was never consummated. On the other hand, for all the allusions to Priscilla as virginal, she had been subjected to significant abuse. What might Westervelt, lacking conscience but possessing an animal nature, have done to her while she was under his control?

16. I believe that Lowe (2017) underestimates the difficulty Zenobia had to surmount: "She casts away the flower just as she casts away Westervelt because they no longer suit her" (p. 72).
17. Priscilla beseeches Zenobia, "Pray do not ask me my other name —at least, not yet—if you will be so kind to a forlorn creature" (p. 29).
18. Harvey L. Gable, Jr. aptly characterizes Zenobia and Priscilla's predicament vis à vis their father: "both sisters are completely dependent on a seedy and malicious beggar for their fortunes, a beggar who is constitutionally incapable of dividing his affections or his money evenly between the two of them" (p. 272).
19. Westervelt, having heard of Priscilla's abilities as a medium, visits heart home and took "advantage of [her]…lack of earthy substance to subject her to himself" (p. 188); thus began Priscilla's bondage to him. At these visits her father "was supposed always to be present" (p. 188). If Old Moodie was indeed present, and not simply negligent, a scenario is created akin to that in *The House of the Seven Gables* when Gervayse Pyncheon is in attendance as Matthew Maule mesmerizes and enslaves his daughter, Alice. Coverdale's narrative does not make clear how Westervelt happened to become involved with both half-sisters.
20. Not all critics agree with my assessment of Priscilla's insubstantiality. Kenneth Kupsh (2004) considers that "There can be little argument that from Coverdale's point of view the story begins and ends with the existence of Priscilla" (p. 3). Later in the essay, the author judges Priscilla to be "the novel's most remarkable and independent personality."
21. Coverdale decenters the reader's focus by entitling the chapter in which there is a rupture in his relationship with Hollingsworth, "A Crisis".
22. Holgrave's "Legend of Alice Pyncheon" in *The House of the Seven Gables* is another instance of the transformation of mental conflict into artistic creation and is discussed in Chapter Three, "' Holgrave's Transformation in *The House of the Seven Gables*: The black moment became at once a blissful one.'"
23. The returned gaze and its significance is creatively explored by David Greven (2012) in his essay "In a Pig's Eye: Masculinity, Mastery and the Returned Gaze of *The Blithedale Romance*".
24. Ullén (2004) suggests that in exchange for Zenobia's cooperation in returning Priscilla to him, Westervelt will agree to grant her a divorce so she is free to marry Hollingsworth (p. 237). Another hypothesis, and one I favor, is that Westervelt threatens to divulge their secret liaison to Hollingsworth, who fancies himself a moralist, but will refrain from doing so if she conspires with him.
25. Old Moodie, temperamental, as his moniker implies, is enraged when he espies, for a moment, Zenobia's dismissive gesture toward Priscilla in response to the young woman's excessive show of affection; Zenobia, unawares, had thwarted the old man's wish, as he expressed to Hollingsworth, to "see that beautiful lady holding my little girl by the hand" (Hawthorne, Vol. 3, p. 87). I do not agree with Ullén that this was the moment that Old Moodie decides with finality to divest Zenobia of her wealth (Ullén, 2004,

p. 217). He may have given voice to this threat which Westervelt somehow heard of and then conveys to Zenobia. It was sometime after his visit to Blithedale that Old Moodie summons Zenobia to his chamber, perhaps motived by an indecision regarding his fortune. He is sufficiently satisfied with her radiant beauty as a reflection of his past glory as to allow her to retain her fortune, for the time being. He issues a warning which intimates his capacity to exercise arbitrary control over her fortune: "Keep it—keep all your wealth—until I demand it all, or none!" (Hawthorne, Vol. 3, p.191). Zenobia ascribes this obscure threat to his being old and deranged.

26. Upon seeing Priscilla with Westervelt in Zenobia's drawing room, Coverdale asks her, "Does Hollingsworth know you are here?" to which she answers, "He bade me come" (p. 171).
27. Zenobia's message to Hollingsworth, "Tell him he has murdered me!" (p. 226) gives vent to her fury and desire for revenge. However, a few minutes earlier she had remarked, "And yet, if he had trusted me, and borne with me a little longer, I would have saved him all this trouble" (p. 225). One wonders if Zenobia is implying that the position into which she had descended was sufficient reason for suicide, even if Hollingsworth had stood by her. Suicide always leaves troubling and unanswerable questions in its wake. As we try to grasp the meanings encoded in all she says to Coverdale in this, her final scene, the reader needs remember that the direness of her situation goes far to account for "the strange way in which her mind seemed to vibrate from the deepest earnest to mere levity" (p. 226). Coverdale, ever alert throughout the romance to intimations of oncoming crisis, is, in the end, insensible to Zenobia's intention. His unconscious, however, reads her strange manner accurately, and, in a dream, will soon warn him of a looming "tragical catastrophe" (p. 228).
28. Dimmesdale's *anagnorisis* and transformation at the end of *The Scarlet Letter* is the subject of Chapter Two.
29. That Hawthorne characterizes Zenobia's action as "bruising herself" constitutes a definitive retort to those who deny she committed suicide. He is, after all, the novel's author.
30. Cited in *The Recognition of Nathaniel Hawthorne* (1969, p. 66). This essay was published anonymously but is almost universally attributed to Eliot. It bears many characteristics of her writing style and artistic values.
31. Mitchell (1998) also concludes that Coverdale is in love with Zenobia: the memory of Zenobia's voice "warns that she cannot be silenced by denial or death but will haunt the heart…He cannot name her, but he can give her a name, and that name is Zenobia" (pp. 203–204).
32. Lowe (2017) remarks that "Though both Coverdale and Zenobia pointedly insist that they would never have fallen in love, we can speculate if Coverdale might have become more than a 'Minor Poet' if they had." (p. 73).
33. The tears that John Marcher sheds for the first time at May Bartram's grave in Henry James's *The Beast in the Jungle*, recall Coverdale's delayed tears of grief for Zenobia.
34. To appreciate the narrow range of Coverdale's feelings for Priscilla, which accords with the slimness of her appeal, the reader need go no further than what is amongst the most anemic professions of love in all literature. Coverdale instructs a bird to convey a message to Priscilla: "And say that, if any mortal really cares for her, it is myself, and not even I, for her realities—poor little seamstress, as Zenobia rightly called her—but for the fancy-work with which I have idly decked her out!" (p. 100). One is embarrassed for the bird.

References

Baym, N. (1968). *The Blithedale Romance*: A Radical Reading. *The Journal of English and Germanic Philology*, *67*.

Beauchamp, G. (2002). Hawthorne and the Universal Reformers. *Utopian Studies*, *13*.

Bell, M. (1962). *Hawthorne's View of the Artist*. New York: University Publishers.

Chodorow, N. J. (1978). *The Reproduction of Mothering: Psychoanalysis and the Sociology of Gender*. Berkeley: University of California Press.

Chodorow, N. J. (1999). *The Power of Feelings*. New Haven: Princeton.

Christophersen, B. (1982). Behind the White Veil: Self-Awareness in Hawthorne's *The Blithedale Romance*. *Modern Language Studies*, *12*.

Cohen, B. B. (Ed.). (1969). *The Recognition of Nathaniel Hawthorne*. Ann Arbor: University of Michigan Press.

Colacurcio, M. (2008). Nobody's Protest Novel: Art and Politics in *The Blithedale Romance*. *Nathaniel Hawthorne Review*, *34*, 1–39.

Crews, F. (1996). *The Sins of the Father: Hawthorne's Psychological Themes*. New York: Oxford University Press.

Dill, E. (2011). Angels of the House, Ghosts of the Commune: Zenobia as Sentimental Woman in *The Blithedale Romance*. *Nathaniel Hawthorne Review*, *37*.

Eliot, G. (1852). Contemporary Literature of America *The Blithedale Romance*. *Westminster Review*, 592–598.

Freud, S. (1959). Mourning and Melancholia. In J. Strachey (Ed.), *The Standard Edition of the Complete Psychological Works of Sigmund Freud* (J. Strachey, Trans., pp. 243–258). Hogarth Press and the Institute of Psycho-Analysis.

Gable, H. Jr. (1994). Unappeasable Longings: Hawthorne, Romance, and the Disintegration of Coverdale's Self in *The Blithedale Romance*. *The New England Quarterly*, *67*, 257–278.

Gates, B. (1988). *Victorian Suicide: Mad Crimes and Sad Histories*. Princeton University Press.

Greven, D. (2012). *The Fragility of Manhood: Hawthorne, Freud and the Politics of Gender*. Columbus: Ohio State University Press.

Hawthorne, N. (1962a). *Blithedale Romance*. In W. Charvat (Ed.), *The Centenary Edition of the Works of Nathaniel Hawthorne* (Vol. 3). Columbus: Ohio State University Press.

Hawthorne, N. (1962b). *The House of the Seven Gables*. In W. Charvat (Ed.), *The Centenary Edition of the Works of Nathaniel Hawthorne* (Vol. 2). Columbus: Ohio University State Press.

Hawthorne, N. (1962c). *The Marble Faun*. In W. Charvat (Ed.), *The Centenary Edition of the Works of Nathaniel Hawthorne* (Vol. 4). Columbus: Ohio State University Press.

Hawthorne, N. (1962d). *The Scarlet Letter*. In W. Charvat (Ed.), *The Centenary Edition of the Works of Nathaniel Hawthorne* (Vol. 1). Columbus: Ohio State University Press.

Hawthorne, N. (1974a). The Hall of Fantasy. In W. Charvat (Ed.), *The Centenary Edition of the Works of Nathaniel Hawthorne* (Vol. 10). Columbus: Ohio State University Press.

Hawthorne, N. (1974b). The Haunted Mind. In W. Charvat (Ed.), *The Centenary Editions of the Works of Nathaniel Hawthorne* (Vol. 9. Columbus: Ohio University State Press.

Hedges, W. (1960). Hawthorne's *Blithedale*: The Function of the Narrator. *Twentieth Century Fiction, 14.*

James, H. (2011). *The Beast in the Jungle.* London: Penguin.

Kupsh, K. (2004). The Modern Tragedy of Blithedale. *Studies in the Novel, 36.*

Kushner, H. I. (1985). Women and Suicide in Historical Perspective. *Signs, 10*(3).

Levy, L. (1968). *The Blithedale Romance*: Hawthorne's 'Voyage Through Chaos'. *Studies in Romanticism, 8.*

Lewis, F. (1992). Women, Death and Theatricality in *The Blithedale Romance. Journal of American Studies, 26.*

Lowe, R. (2017). Free Love Among the Ruins. *Nathaniel Hawthorne Review, 43*(1).

Male, R. R. (1957). *Hawthorne's Tragic Vision.* New York: W.W. Norton.

Matheson, T. (1976). Feminism and Femininity in *The Blithedale Romance. Nathaniel Hawthorne Journal, 48,* 215–226.

Matthiessen, F. O. (1941). *American Renaissance: Art and Expression in the Age of Emerson and Whitman.* New York: Oxford University Press.

McElroy, J., & McDonald, E. (1982). The Coverdale Romance. *Studies in the Novel, 14.*

Miller, J. (2000). Eros and Ideology: at the Heart of Hawthorne's *Blithedale. Nineteenth Century Literature, 8.*

Millington, R. H. (1992). *Practicing Romance: Narrative Form and Cultural Engagement in Hawthorne's Fiction.* Princeton: Princeton University Press.

Mills, A. (2003). 'The Sweet Word,' Sister: The Transformative Threat of Sisterhood and *The Blithedale Romance. ATQ, 17.*

Mitchell, T. (1998). *Hawthorne's Fuller Mystery.* Amherst: University of Massachusetts Press.

Pfister, J. (1991). *The Production of Personal Life: Class, Gender, and the Psychological in Hawthorne's Fiction.* Stanford University Press.

Schriber, M. (1982). Justice to Zenobia. *The New England Quarterly, 55.*

Ullén, M. (2004). *The Half-Vanished Structure: Hawthorne's Allegorical Dialectics.* Bern: Peter Lang.

Wagenknecht, E. (1989). *Nathaniel Hawthorne: The Man, His Tales and Romances.* New York: Continuum.

Ware, W. (1838). *Zenobia or The Fall of Palmyra.* C.S. Francis.

Wordsworth, W. (1798). *Lines Composed a Few Miles above Tintern Abbey, On Revisiting the Banks of the Wye during a Tour. July 13, 1798.* Retrieved from Poetry Foundation www.poetryfoundation.org/poems/45527/lines-composed-a-few-miles-above-tintern-abbey-on-revisiting-the-banks-of-the-wye-during-a-tour-july-13-1798.

5 Miriam's Transformation in *The Marble Faun*: "The tragic dignity of their hour of crime"

The murder of the Model is the central event around which *The Marble Faun* is structured: all aspects of the narrative converge toward it and radiate from it. "Fatal chance" has brought Miriam and the Model together in the Catacomb of Saint Calixtus, an encounter which sets them on a trajectory to calamity (Hawthorne, 1962, Vol. 4, p. 95). After seeing Miriam again, the Model's erotic obsession is reignited and it drives him to shadow her relentlessly. When he overtakes her in the Borghese Grove, he makes clear his intention to possess her: she must soon flee Rome with him or he will exercise his power over her and destroy her new life. As he is deaf to pleas to leave her in peace, Miriam reminds her persecutor: "I foresee the end, and have already warned you of it. It will be death!" (p. 97). On the moonlight ramble, she senses danger in Donatello's increasing rage toward the Model and she exhorts him: "Peace, peace, Donatello...Do him no mischief!" (p. 148). Despite Miriam's efforts to avert it, in a moment of overpowering instinctual force, the calamity is enacted. As the Model takes steps toward her on a terrace overlooking the precipice, Miriam's statement, uttered earlier that night, proves to have been prophetic: "The firmest substance of human happiness is but a thin crust spread over it...It needs no earthquake to open the chasm. A footstep, a little heavier than ordinary, will serve...to break through the crust, at any moment. By-and-by, we inevitably sink!" (pp. 162–163).

With the resounding thump of the Model's body issuing up from the base of the Tarpeian Rock, Death, the immitigable instructor in all Hawthorne's romances, commences its stern office. Nina Baym (1971) aptly judges that "Coming to terms with this killing is, for the readers as well as the characters, the main business of the romance" (p. 356). Indeed, that catastrophic moment serves as a catalyst to crucial transformations in all four protagonists which unfold in the second half of the romance, thereby justifying Hawthorne's choice of *Transformation* as the novel's title for its first publication in England. During Carnival, Kenyon, remembering their celebration the year before, reflects: "We are all so changed!" (Hawthorne, 1962, Vol. 4, p. 427).

Donatello's violent action determines his abrupt fall from innocence and initiates a painful journey through punishing guilt to virtuous love and repentance. The narrator takes note that "the faun's transformation" (Hawthorne, 1962, Vol. 4, p. 172) begins with this act: "fierce energy had… kindled him into a man and developed within him an intelligence…But that simple and joyous creature was gone forever" (p. 172). Kenyon's two busts of Donatello are attempts to capture the transformation in sculpture. Hilda, having observed a murder which was provoked by her closest friend, implodes psychologically and falls into a state of depression in which she loses interest in what had been her all-consuming artistic passion. Her mounting torment, bringing her to the brink of insanity, breaks down her self-sufficiency; the vulnerabilities that are therein exposed ready her for a stabilizing romantic attachment to the sculptor.[1] Kenyon, although not a direct participant in the murder scene, correctly intuits its contours and derives mutative knowledge and wisdom in his crucial role as trusted counselor to his deeply troubled friends. Hilda's disappearance, time-limited though it proves to be, leaves him depleted of artistic will; the desolation he experiences without her prepares him to embrace both the felicities and compromises that an enduring bond with her will entail.

The full weight of the consequences of the scene's impact on Donatello as well as on Hilda, however, fall heavily upon Miriam for her part in inciting it; how she deals with this burden defines the woman that she is and brings with it the most significant transformation in the romance, one which lies at the emotional core of the romance. As I will detail, from the victim of trauma, desperately seeking freedom from a tyrant and long alienated from love and sympathy, she emerges as a woman of high moral stature, with deep insight into life's mysteries and a capacity for generous love although it involves sacrifice and irredeemable loss. This psychological transformation which imbues Miriam with tragic dignity is the subject of the essay's inquiry which presents that first systematic analysis of Miriam's psychology in the critical literature. Although the Model's murder is widely appreciated as pivotal to the plot, its crucial place in the vicissitudes of Miriam's psychological development has not been rigorously explored.

It is a fiendish irony that Miriam's formidable resources of intelligence and force of character abandon her at the verge of disaster. After months of persecution and efforts to free herself from it, the moment of chaos brings with it conflicts which overwhelm her psychological resources and precipitate a lapse of consciousness in the form of a depersonalized state. As the Model draws near the edge of the precipice "a sick despair crept over her that impeded her breath and benumbed her natural promptitude of thought. Miriam seemed dreamily to remember falling on her knees; but, in her whole recollection of that wild moment, she beheld herself as in a dim show, and could not well distinguish what was done and suffered; no, not even whether she was really an actor and sufferer in the scene" (p. 171). Through this lapse of consciousness, Miriam's psychological defenses protect her from the pain of participation in the existential terror of the moment. However, without the controls that inhere in consciousness, she falls prey to the power of the unconscious.

In his early sketch, "The Haunted Mind" (1835), Hawthorne adumbrates Miriam's situation: "In the depths of every heart, there is a tomb and a dungeon, though the lights, the music, and revelry above may cause us to forget their existence, and the buried ones, or prisoners whom they hide. But sometimes, and oftenest at midnight, those dark receptacles are flung wide open" (Vol. 9, pp. 201–202). In the extremity of the moment, the portals of Miriam's haunted mind are flung open, and the buried ones that emerged are accurately identified by Hilda in her friend's eyes: "A look of hatred, triumph, vengeance, and, as it were, joy at some unhoped for relief!" (p. 210).[2]

Using this eruption of the unconscious as the focus of inquiry, I will apply a psychoanalytic lens to Miriam's history and character in order to elucidate the dynamics of this critical moment and the transformation that result from it. By using insights derived from the analysis, I will attempt to reconstruct the gaps of Miriam's memory as well as her part as "actor and sufferer" in the scene. I will conclude that the Model's relentless pursuit of her re-enacts the drama of his erotic compulsion toward her in her childhood, which she relives during the moonlight ramble with mounting dread and panic. Alone and unprotected as a child, she was the Model's powerless victim; protest and rage against him were repressed. Trapped, as it were, on the edge of the Tarpeian Rock, Miriam is forced to re-experience the climax of a once familiar desperation. However, this time a champion appears in the form of Donatello who puts into action her repressed wish to take revenge on her nemesis and be freed of him forever. Donatello's devotion and selfless action, fulfilling her childhood longing to be protected by a father, penetrate longstanding emotional defenses and are gratefully received into her heart. The moment of chaotic violence serves as a reparative of childhood trauma and, with the same stroke, ushers Miriam into the enchantment of love. It is the essence of her tragic fate that the decisive act that brings Miriam a man to love and protect her creates the consequence by which she loses him forever.

Whose Miriam

Augustus M. Kolish (2001) remarks on the mist of uncertainty that has long surrounded readings of Miriam: "For over a hundred years, Hawthorne's coyness about Miriam's past has provoked puzzlement and unanswered questions among the story's readers...At the center of Miriam's characterization lies one of the greatest mysteries in Hawthorne's fiction: who was she? What was the crime that compels her to seek anonymity in Rome? And from where did this 'likeable criminal'... emerge?" (p. 431). Hawthorne's narrative strategy of delaying the fullest account of Miriam's life until practically the end of the novel indeed complicates settling questions about her. As with the discovery in the closing pages of *The House of the Seven Gables* that Holgrave is a Maule, the reader of *The Marble Faun* is compelled to re-index what is known about Miriam in light of new and crucial information about her past divulged to Kenyon on the Campagna. For Elissa Greenwald (1991), at least, this information "comes too late in the story to account for its emotional effects" (p. 136). I would propose, instead, that Hawthorne is adhering to a rigorous aesthetic standard for works of art, expressed by Hilda: "'Their highest merit is suggestiveness'" (Hawthorne, 1962, Vol. 4, p. 379).[3] The narrator concurs: "A picture, however admirable the painter's art, and wonderful his power, requires of the spectator a surrender of himself...There is always the necessity of helping out the painter's art with our own resources of sensibility and imagination" (p. 335). Everything that Hilda and the narrator say about pictorial art is equally true of a literary romance. Nowhere is the reader's participation more crucial than regarding Miriam. I agree with Gordon Hutner's (1988) assertion: "In leaving key facts indeterminate, Hawthorne means to prod the reader's unpursued possibilities of understanding" (p. 165). To the psychoanalyst, whose mode of collecting data relies significantly on suggestiveness, *The Marble Faun* offers abundant information about the conscious and unconscious aspects of Miriam's emotional life. In my estimation, she is among the most fully realized and complex characters in Hawthorne's oeuvre. The inferences and the interpretations that I offer are based on this data and inform the construction of a psychological narrative of substantial explanatory power. A psychoanalytic reading of her character accords with Baym's (1971) conclusion that "despite its agitated rhetoric, *The Marble Faun* has a driving unity and a surprisingly straightforward narrative line" (p. 355).

Given Richard H. Millington's (1992) astute judgment that *The Marble Faun* is an extended exploration of the "imperium of conscience," (p. 177) it is surprising to discover the paucity of systematic commentaries about Miriam's psychology. What the narrator says about her early in the romance perhaps predicts what would be true of critics' responses to her: "She resembled one of those images of light which conjurors evoke and cause to shine before us, in apparent tangibility, only at an arm's length beyond our grasp; we make a step in advance, expecting to seize the illusion, but find it still precisely far out of our reach" (Hawthorne, 1962, Vol. 4, p. 21).

In a book-length treatment of *The Marble Faun* (1992), Evan Carton does not explore Hawthorne's handling of the characters' psychology. He does underscore one aspect of Miriam's psychology in the supposition that she "has violently resisted or revolted against a powerful figure of male authority, probably a rapacious father," (p. 91) and speculates further that her artistic work is "the product of certain complex personal relations to gender roles that are deeply engrained in and powerfully reinforced by the larger society" (p. 126). Carton is concerned with Miriam's emotional life to the extent that her dilemma reveals the author's unresolved cultural conflicts. We can gauge how far the guiding principle of literary criticism has shifted from that of New Criticism in Carton's candid conclusion: "*The Marble Faun* is most interesting, from this standpoint, not as a vehicle of human wisdom, nor as an object in and of itself, but as an accessible and vivid site of Hawthorne's lifelong struggle, and of the struggle of the American culture at an important moment in its development with the psychology and politics of gender"

(p. 126). Frederick Crews (1966), in a widely-quoted psychoanalytic study, is more interested in Miriam as symptomatic of what he sees as Hawthorne's neurosis than in understanding the complex dynamics of her mind. For Crews, Hawthorne's sexual ambivalence is manifest in the choice between Miriam, "an overblown, oversexed, aggressive woman," and Hilda, "a fragile, childlike, impregnable and impenetrable maiden" (p. 215). Crews's inaccurate characterizations of both women are freighted with harsh personal judgments. Nor does Miriam's sensuality belong to her but represents for him "the scapegoat for a sexual nausea that Hawthorne, along with his other characters, prefer to vent upon a foreign temptress and her sensual race" (p. 222).[4] Rudolph Von Abele (1955) judges Miriam as an "'amateur'" (p. 90) artist of shallow commitment because she finds "no further necessity of producing art-works once she has beaten down the dragon of sexual temptation by having Donatello kill the model" (p. 90).[5] For Crews, Miriam is Hawthorne's sexual scapegoat, and according to Von Abele, Donatello is Miriam's. On the other hand, Newton Arvin's (1961) unaccountably severe assessment robs Miriam's sensual appeal of any substance: "Miriam is a melodramatic shadow with whom only a faun like Donatello could fall passionately in love, and for whose sake it is somewhat remarkable that even he could commit a crime" (p. 259).

For other critics, Miriam does not possess full personhood, but is apprehended as a projected part of someone else. For example, in reference to the scenes at Monte Beni, Baym (1971) finds that "Miriam, in this part of the book, is less a character than an exiled part of Donatello's being" (p. 364). I would argue that in the crucial scene in The Marble Saloon, Miriam is in full possession of her self. Moreover, while ignoring the exceptional pathos of their mutual farewell at Carnival, Baym judges that in relation to Hilda's release: "Miriam and Donatello both are less whole characters than fragments of Kenyon's exploded psyche" (p. 364).

Ullén's (2004) allegorical analysis of *The Marble Faun*, brilliant though it is, reduces Hawthorne's intricate rendering of psychological transformations to epiphenomena: "the governing principal of the romance cannot primarily be understood as any form of psychological mimesis, but is grounded in purely aesthetic considerations" (p. 278). He asserts that "Hawthorne has very little interest in making his characters conform to the psychological mould that we associate with the realistic novel…Therefore it is crucial that we do not reduce Hilda –or any other of the…characters that people *The Marble Faun*—to representation of a person, but recognize her as the allegorical embodiment of an abstract idea" (p. 287). Ullén caps his argument with a claim that disorients a psychoanalyst: "Like Donatello (and Miriam and Kenyon to a lesser extent), Hilda is not so much a person as a discursive prism" (p. 278). In the Preface to *The House of the Seven Gables*, Hawthorne (1962) allows the romancer "a certain latitude, both as to fashion and material," not enjoyed by a novelist, regarding a "very minute fidelity…to the very course of man's experience" (Vol. 2, p. 1). However, if, as Ullén contends, the characters were not meant to be read essentially as persons, Hawthorne (1962) needs judge that *The*

Marble Faun did "sin unpardonably" in its wide "swerve aside from the truth of the human heart" (Vol. 2, p.1).

Although I do not agree with his understanding of the origin of Miriam's guilt, Spencer Hall's appreciation of Miriam's heroic stature (1970) conforms with mine: "The nature of Miriam's past remains in shadow, but she does succeed in understanding and accepting her own guilt for the murder of the model...and not until she comes to full consciousness of the 'hatred, triumph, vengeance and joy at some hoped for relief' which welled in own heart and which motivated her action can she begin to reaffirm, through penitence, her tragic yet heroic humanity" (p. 93).

This brief survey of some commentary on Miriam is a reminder of the interpretive challenge that *The Marble Faun* famously represents. In an interesting essay on what he calls "monological readings" of Hawthorne's last romance, Michael Dunne (2004) argues against the limitations imposed by a critic's employing one interpretive vantage as it involves "tearing the web apart by sorting through the text...for passages useful in sustaining the critic's monological reading," while suppressing others (p. 26). As a result, Dunne humorously observes, "nearly every critic who writes about *The Marble Faun* has a good idea of what the book 'means' and nearly everyone disagrees about what that meaning is" (p. 25). This psychoanalytic study, alas, is an example of what Dunne urges a critic to eschew, as rather than seeking integrative choral harmony, it will add yet another solo voice to *The Marble Faun's* interpretive cacophony. Will and Mimosa Stephenson's (1995) illuminating study of the "inconspicuous ubiquity" of oxymorons in the text, and they count well over four hundred, suggests to me that Hawthorne employed this rhetorical device not only to gather a cumulative thematic force, but also to create a reading experience which fosters openness to emotional and moral complexity, contradiction and confusion.[6] The range of interpretations to which *The Marble Faun* has been the subject may in part be a result of an existential dislocation that the act of reading it induces. This phenomenology is explored by Sylvie Mathé (1992) in her outstanding essay on the crucial place of oxymorons in *The Scarlet Letter*: "the way to find a bearing on oxymoron can only be to take it in and let it overtake you, to allow its unresolved tensions to work through. The paradoxical nature of oxymoron lies at the root of its subversive impact while the poetic violence which it imposes on language by its explosive pull accounts for its compelling hold" (p. 626).[7]

Freudian psychoanalytic theory, which views the human psyche as always seeking compromise in the face of irreducible conflict within itself, is congenial to the psychological universe of the oxymoron. The narrative of Miriam that I have constructed relies on what Nancy J. Chodorow (1999) designates as psychoanalysis's unique epistemology founded on "the power of feelings," and employs the psychoanalytic method in the service of unraveling "the particularistic uniqueness of each individual psyche and life history" (p. 2). The affinities between Hawthorne and Freud's understanding of the unconscious allow a psychoanalytically-informed narrative, perhaps uniquely, to bring into coherence the romance's elusiveness about Miriam and to offer, in its distinctive voice, an answer to Kolish's (2001) question regarding the mystery that she has posed: "who is she?"

Miriam

Unbeknownst to the reader, by the time of the opening scene in the Capitoline sculpture gallery, the Model's maleficent presence has loomed over Miriam for several months. The Model's determination to be "nothing but a shadow behind your footsteps" (Hawthorne, 1962, Vol. 4, p. 31) results in Miriam's mounting desperation as a woman who is pursued and threatened. Thus, the Miriam introduced to us in the opening chapters is at all times under great psychological duress; the narrator comments on its consequences: "...her happiness was very seriously compromised. Her spirits were often depressed into deep melancholy...She grew moody, moreover, and subject to fits of passionate ill-temper" (p. 35). In despair, she contemplates suicide: "Would not poison make an end of me? Will not the Tiber drown me?" (p. 94).

In order to understand her fate, it is important to appreciate the person she was before the reappearance of the Model so darkened her being. One can, from various sources in the text, assemble a picture of Miriam that shows her to be endowed with extraordinary character and abilities.

Fleeing a scandal involving a crime of which she was innocent, Miriam establishes herself, under new identity, as artist in Rome. This is a bold and courageous step for a woman alone: "she flung herself upon the world, and speedily created a new sphere" (p. 431). Miriam was, in Kenyon's informed estimation, "a proud and self-dependent woman" (p. 283). A connoisseur of fine art, who offers incisive judgments on a variety of masterpieces in Rome, she also comments on works she viewed in the galleries in Naples, the Uffizi, and the Louvre. We do not know about her training or experience as a painter before her arrival in Rome; in any case, her "pictures met with good acceptance among the patrons of modern art" (p. 20) and were admired for their "warmth and passionateness" (p. 20). The narrator's discriminating eye finds much to praise in the works Donatello sees in her studio. He has particular approbation for her genre scenes of domestic life: "feeling and sympathy in all of them were deep and true...they were the productions of a beautiful imagination, dealing with the warm and pure suggestions of a woman's heart" and revealed an impressive "force and variety of imaginative sympathies" (p. 46).

Miriam's "mobile imagination" (p. 78) also finds expression in narrative flights as a story-teller. In response to her friends' questions about the Model, she cleverly deflects their inquiries by letting "her fancy run into wilder fables than any which German ingenuity or Italian superstition had contrived" (pp. 33–34). On another occasion, out of "the exuberance of fancy that distinguished her" (p. 462), Miriam had improvised a "mythical and magical legend" (p. 462) about the gems in her Etruscan bracelet, the memory of which will have enduring significance for Hilda.

Although there is but one mention of it, Miriam was a singer of unusual endowment. The song she sings from below the battlements of Monte Beni, with a voice of "melancholy richness" (p. 269) and an enormous expressive range, moves both Donatello and Kenyon to tears. Her song has resonated with the cords of the human heart which inspires the narrator to offer lavish praise: "Never was there a profounder pathos than breathed through the mysterious voice" (p. 269).[8]

Miriam was an educated woman, as familiar with the history of ancient Rome as with the novels of Mme. de Stael. She had a "natural promptitude of thought" (p. 171) and was considered by Kenyon to possess "high intellectual endowment" (p. 105) and by Hilda to be "so accomplished and gifted" (p. 105). Her personality, albeit "impressible and impulsive," (p. 83) was distinguished by a "woman's kindly charm" (p. 78) as well as an "uprightness and impulsive generosity" (p. 206). Miriam's "personal magnetism" (p. 36) drew to her the friendship of an exacting Hilda who professes, "I love her dearly and trust her most entirely" (p. 108). Kenyon's beautiful words about her to Donatello in Perugia, practically a paean, distill the qualities that I have just detailed: "She has rich gifts of heart and mind, a suggestive power, a magnetic influence, a sympathetic knowledge, which, wisely and religiously exercised, are what your condition needs" (p. 321). Donatello's simpler formula goes to the heart of the matter of Miriam's appeal: "...you are yourself... that is why I love you" (p. 79).

I leave for last Miriam's physical attributes which tend to overwhelm the conversation about her and prompt us to forget her other outstanding qualities. That said, she was of "singular beauty" (p. 279) which invariably contributed to her "large and bounteous impression" (p. 23). There was "an artful beauty in her motion" (p. 85) and Kenyon had long wished to model "that most beautiful and expressive face" (p. 121). Donatello was first taken in by "a beauty which Miriam possessed in a remarkable degree" (p. 22). In an extraordinary attestation, which speaks to his, too, having fallen under her irresistible allure, the narrator describes in Miriam's self-portrait "a beautiful woman, such as one sees only two or three times, if even so many in all a lifetime; so beautiful, that she seemed to get into your consciousness and memory, and could never afterwards be shut out, but haunted your dreams, for pleasure or for pain; holding your inner realm as a conquered territory, though without deigning to make herself at home there" (pp. 47–48).[9]

With regard to the Model, such beauty is a curse and not a blessing. After re-encountering Miriam in the catacomb, the Model again yields his inner realm to her, as it were, and as the monomaniacal compulsion to possess her attests, despite prayers and penance, he is thereafter powerless to shut her out.[10] The Model revisits the pleasure and pain of this erotic thrall by inflicting sadistic domination on its source. After catching a glimpse of a beseeching Miriam kneeling to the Model in the public glare of the Piazza del Popolo, Kenyon has a telling fantasy: "Free as she seemed to be—beggar as he looked—the nameless vagrant must then be dragging the beautiful

Miriam through the streets of Rome, fettered and shackled more cruelly than any captive queen of yore, following in an Emperour's triumph" (p. 108).

Although the community of artists and her friends are perplexed by the Model's attachment to Miriam, they ascribe it to the magnetic nature of her beauty which attracts untoward male attention, a not uncommon hazard, both then and now, for a beautiful woman on the streets of Rome.[11] They view his stalking her with bemused interest; only Donatello instinctually reacts, with "invincible repugnance" (p. 90), to the threat that the Model poses to Miriam. No one knows, and Miriam keeps it secret, that her relationship with the Model has deep and poisonous roots, both in her recent past and in her childhood: "The spectral figure she encountered there [the Catacomb] was the Evil Fate that had haunted her through life" (p. 432).

Miriam and the Model

In their turbulent interchange in the Borghese Grove, the Model is first to mention knowing Miriam when she was a child: "These many months of trouble" which he visited upon her and which he concedes constitutes the "later thraldom in which I hold you... [have] scarcely made your cheek paler than I saw in your childhood, Miriam" (p. 94). That he specifies her face, an aspect of her physical being, is significant. His part in her childhood is further elaborated when she gazes at his corpse in the Church of the Cappuchini: "Yes; these were the features that [she] had known so well; this was the visage that she remembered from far longer date than the most intimate of her friends suspected" (p. 190). Nor was this a happy recollection: his dead form "held the evil spirit which blasted her sweet youth, and compelled her, as it were, to stain her womanhood with crime" (p. 190). The verb "blasted" suggests that she was a victim of violent or destructive action. The narrator subtly alludes to a physical relationship between them in the observation that Miriam "bent down over the dead monk, till one of her rich curls brushed against his forehead. She touched one of his folded hands with her finger" (p. 191). The identity of the corpse is confirmed by its bearing a physical mark, a scar: "It is he!...There is the scar that I know so well on his brow" (p. 191). The use of the term, "blasted," and the attention they both pay to what is familiar in each other's bodies, are instances of the "highest merit of suggestiveness" (p. 379) leading to an interpretation, developed below, that Miriam was the victim of childhood abuse by the Model.

Miriam eventually reveals crucial information about her childhood to Kenyon, which sets the context for further analysis of her psychology. Her mother was of English descent, "with a vein... of Jewish blood" (p. 429), and died when Miriam was a child. Such a loss is always traumatic, and all the more so because of the dangers that Miriam was left to contend with on her own. She joins Hester and Zenobia as Hawthorne heroines whose intimate life goes awry without the protective guidance of a mother. It is noteworthy that we hear nothing about Miriam's father except that he was from a prominent family in south Italy. Instead, Miriam tells Kenyon about a relative of her father, "a certain marchese" (p. 430), who arranged a contract of betrothal to her when she was just a child. This was arrangement "between two persons of disproportionate ages, and in which feelings went for nothing" (p. 430).[12] In fact, Miriam was forcefully against this union. Through an extraordinary act of will, and drawing on an identification with her deceased mother's strength, she was eventually able to prevent it. Whatever her comprehension of the *marchese* when she was young, her judgment of his character looking back was chillingly negative: "he betrayed traits so *evil*, so treacherous, so wild, and yet so strangely *subtle*, as could only be accounted for by...*insanity*" (p. 430, emphases added).

The similarity between Miriam's characterization of the *marchese* and the following description by the narrator of the Model implies that they are the same person: "there seemed to be a mysterious fascination in the influence of this ill-omened person over Miriam; it was such as beasts and reptiles, of *evil and subtle nature*, sometimes exercise over their victims" (p. 93, emphasis added). Miriam believes that the marchese suffered from insanity and she also concludes that the Model's "very acts of depravity" (p. 432), indicate that "*insanity* must have been mixed up with his original composition" (p. 430, emphasis added). She instructs Donatello: "Do him no mischief! He is mad; and we are as mad as he is, if we suffer ourselves to be disquieted by his antics" (p. 95). Therefore what she says over the Model's dead body is also her judgment of him as the *marchese*, her childhood betrothed: "There was nothing, in this lifetime, viler than this man. She knew it; there was no other fact within her consciousness that she felt to be so certain" (p. 191). Her tortuous attachment to him, which spanned the early bondage of her childhood and her "later thraldom" to him for months in Rome, had been "forged in some unhallowed furnace as is only kindled by evil passions and fed by evil deeds" (p. 93). These are the passions and deeds which had surely "blasted her sweet childhood" (p. 190). In Rome the Model engages in pursuit, threat and intimidation; the earlier thraldom, more damaging because it was inflicted on her as a child, undoubtedly involved similar malevolent behavior. In order to understand the "prisoners" released from Miriam's haunted mind, we must identify the "evil passions" and the "very acts of depravity" that she was victimized by in her childhood. In this inquiry, the reader benefits from the "great merit of suggestiveness" offered by the central position Hawthorne accords the story of Beatrice Cenci in the inner workings of *The Marble Faun*.

Hilda's Beatrice Cenci

It is no accident that the new work that Hilda unveils to Miriam upon her visit to her studio is a copy of Guido Reni's portrait of Beatrice Cenci. Given the superabundance of religious art in Rome, it is an odd choice of subject for a saintly woman such as Hilda. However, with her exquisite sensitivity, which operates beneath awareness, I believe that Hilda was drawn to Guido's work because it portrays a central feature of her dear friend's troubled soul. That is, Guido's Beatrice Cenci, in her look of sorrow and isolation, resonated with Hilda's experience of Miriam, and the artist in her unconsciously sought a means to express it pictorially. The narrator comments on the quality of sorrow of Hilda's Beatrice: "It was a sorrow that removed this beautiful girl out of the sphere of humanity, and set her in a far-off region, the remoteness of which...makes us shiver as at a spectre" (p. 64). Kenyon and Hilda sense a sorrow of this kind in an emotionally distant Miriam who "might stretch out her hand and never clasp a hand of [her friends]...This perception of an infinite, shivering solitude, amid which we cannot come close enough to human beings to be warmed by them...is one of the most forlorn results of an accident, misfortune, crime or peculiarity, that puts an individual ajar with the world" (p. 113). We see Miriam put ajar at the height of her unconstrained participation in a sylvan dance when the Model appears next to her and "a strange distance and unapproachableness had all at once enveloped her" (p. 89).

What, then, is the relationship between Miriam's misfortune and that of Beatrice Cenci? Beatrice, as history and legend have it, was raped by her infamously cruel father; because the Papal authority refused to take action against him, she participated in a family plot and assassinated him, for which all involved were convicted and executed. Guido's portrait was said to be painted in Beatrice's prison cell while she was awaiting execution. In his Italian journal, Hawthorne records the unique impact of the portrait: "It is the very saddest picture that was ever painted or conceived; there is an unfathomable depth and sorrow in the eyes; the sense of it comes to you by a sort of intuition...It is the most profoundly wrought picture in the world; no artist did it, or could do it again" (Gollin, 1975, p. 2). However, for all the evocativeness of the painting, I believe that Hawthorne was more influenced by his reading of a literary rendering of Beatrice's story, namely, Shelley's verse play, *The Cenci* (1819).[13] In the Preface, Shelley records, in terms which Hawthorne will later echo, his captivation with Guido's painting, in which he finds: "a simplicity and dignity which united with the exquisite loveliness and deep sorrow are inexpressibly pathetic" (p. 7).

In *The Cenci*, Shelley invests the characters in this horrific family drama with what he imagined to be their thoughts and feelings. He states and his purpose in the Preface: "...such a story, if told so as to present to the reader all the feelings of those who acted in it, their hopes and fears, their confidences and misgivings, their various passions, and opinions, acting upon and with each other, yet all conspiring to one tremendous end, would be as a light to make apparent some of the most dark and secret caverns of the human heart" (Shelley, p. 3). We discern resonances of Shelley's design in Hawthorne's effort to illuminate the secrets of Miriam's mind in its relation to her tormented bond to the Model. In language that recalls Shelley's, Miriam asks: "Is the dark dream, in which I walk, of such solid, stony substance, that there can be no escape out of its dungeon?" (Hawthorne, 1962, Vol. 4, p. 82). As if in response, the narrator remarks, "if her soul was apt to lurk in the darkness of a cavern, she could sport madly in the sunshine before the cavern's mouth" (p. 83).

As a noteworthy instance of intertextuality, I believe that Hawthorne absorbed Shelley's imagining of the interior world of Beatrice and invested it in Miriam. Therefore, a study of Shelley's Beatrice can shed light on Miriam's psychological narrative. Cenci foresaw that the rape of his daughter would be: "A deed which shall confound both night and day…'. Tis she shall grope through a bewildering mist of horror: if there be a sun in heaven she shall not dare to look upon its beams; nor feel its warmth" (p. 27, lines 183–187). Like Beatrice, Miriam will also find herself cut off from sources of warmth, as she inhabits: "an infinite, shivering solitude, amid which we cannot come close enough to human beings to be warmed by them" (Hawthorne, 1962, Vol. 4, p. 113). The Model's "very acts of depravity" resonate with Cenci's violation of his daughter which "dissolves [her] flesh to a pollution, poisoning the subtle, pure and inmost spirit of life!" (Shelley, p. 33, lines 21–23). The trauma brings Beatrice close to insanity: "My God! I never knew what the mad felt before: for I am mad beyond all doubt!" (p. 33, lines 24–25). Beatrice does not keep her violation secret; whatever acts of depravity Miriam suffered, the secret she keeps about them results in near emotional collapse. She admits to Kenyon "There is a secret in my heart that burns me! –that tortures me! Sometimes, I fear to go mad of it!" (Hawthorne, 1962, Vol. 4, p. 128). When the trauma of rape strains Beatrice's psyche to the breaking point, she enters into a state of depersonalization in which she can no longer discern reality from fantasy: "I thought I was that wretched Beatrice men speak of, whom her father sometimes hauls from hall to hall by the entangled hair; and other, pens up naked in damp cells…this wofull story so did I overact in my sick dreams, that I imagine…no, it cannot be!" (p. 34, lines 43–50). As discussed earlier, at the Tarpeian Rock, Miriam's psyche also defends itself by removing her into a similarly dissociated mental state: "she beheld herself as in a dim show, and could not well distinguish what was done and suffered" (p. 171).

There is a crucial moral ambiguity with which both *The Cenci and The Marble Faun* struggle. With no hope of Papal intervention, Beatrice's fiancé, Giocomo, adopts a position that Beatrice's plan to murder Cenci "turns black parricide to piety" (p. 70. lines 44–45). Standing in front of Hilda's portrait of Beatrice, Miriam voices the possibility of a similar moral judgment: "Beatrice's sin may not have been so great; perhaps it was not sin at all but the best virtue possible in the circumstances" (Hawthorne, 1962, Vol. 4, p. 66), a question that Kenyon will later echo in relation to the murder of the Model.

Beatrice was not only raped by her father when she was a woman, but was also a victim of abuse in childhood, as she laments: "And so my lot was ordered, that a father first turned the moments of awakening life to drops, each poisoning youth's sweet hope and then stabbed with one blow my everlasting soul; and my untainted fame" (p. 77, lines 121–125) the "moments of awakening life" refer to her childhood; she was "stabbed with one blow" when raped in the course of the play. Like Beatrice, Miriam was the victim of domination and abuse by a paternal figure both as a child and an adult.

Miriam, looking deeply into Hilda's portrait, sees herself in Beatrice; in a significant sense, this tells us as much as we need to know. Miriam is also speaking of herself when she avows: "Beatrice's own conscience does not acquit her of something evil, and never to be forgiven" (Hawthorne, 1962, Vol. 4, p. 66). However unjustified, a victim of abuse always bears a darkened conscience as part of its legacy. Through her identification with Beatrice, Miriam believes she sees her more fully than even Guido could: "If a woman had painted the original picture, there might have been something in it which we miss now. I have a great mind to undertake a copy myself, and try to give it what it lacks" (p. 68). *The Cenci* gives Beatrice a platform to reveal the brutal confinement, physical abuse, and rape by her father. Shelley is graphic; Hawthorne is allusive. What the Model/*marchese* had done to Miriam in the past is left to the reader's imagination, which Hawthorne colors through associations to Beatrice's story. However, we can say with authority that the Model's erotic monomania, so urgent toward Miriam as a woman, when directed at her as a child, with or without actual physical violation, effected significant emotional trauma upon her. A child's psyche, needing safety and security in parental affection, cannot bear the weight of sexual attention for the purpose of the adult's gratification, which constitutes a perversion of the parental role. The psychoanalytic literature from Freud onward documents the adverse psychological consequences of such attention to the child in the form of a variety of neurotic symptoms, including anxiety, depression, guilt, self-loathing, sexual inhibition, isolation, helplessness, and rage. The contemporary psychoanalyst, Leonard Shengold (1989), has suitably termed the systematic abuse of a child, "soul murder" (p. 19).[14] As the Model closes in on her, thereby evoking disturbing feelings from her past, Miriam evidences a number of these sequelae of trauma. I mention one in particular: early in the novel, Miriam makes light of Donatello's declaration that he would be happy with her forever. She exclaims, "The child!—the simpleton!" (p. 81). Moments later, however, "her eyes filled with tears" as she felt "this zephyr of a new affection, with its untainted freshness, blow over her weary, stifled heart, which had no right to be revived by it. The very exquisiteness of the enjoyment made her know that it ought to be a forbidden one" (p. 82). For Miriam, even a hint of sensual pleasure signals the need for repression and indicates that the superego will repudiate any gratification of the id. A confused sense of guilt for being the object of a parent's sexual arousal results in a drive for self-punishment, and is one of the most unfortunate and enduring consequences of childhood sexual abuse. Kenyon senses constraints of this sort in his observation about Miriam: "and even now she is imprisoned there in a kind of cage the iron bars of which are made of her own thought" (p. 112). Miriam's emotional entrapment is also manifest in her sketches of family life, where she represents herself as a voyeur to scenes of family intimacy, from which she is excluded: "In all these sketches of common life...a figure was pourtrayed apart…and always depicted with an expression of deep sadness; and in every instance, slightly as they were brought out, the face and form had the traits of Miriam's own" (p. 46).

That Terrible Event

Although Miriam evades marriage to the Model, she was not free of him thereafter. Given his obsession with her, it is likely that he could not long restrain himself from pursuing her. What he says to Miriam later in the Borghese Grove expresses an unshakable conviction that must have long held sway: "We have a destiny, which we must needs fulfill together" (p. 94). The narrator reports that with the marriage plan thwarted, "Some time afterward had occurred that terrible event…the frightening and mysterious circumstances of which will recur to many minds" (p. 231). Although neither Miriam nor the narrator is explicit about it, it is possible for the reader to adduce a credible narrative of what transpired. The "terrible event," I imagine, involved a murder perpetrated by the Model against a man who he perceived to be a rival for Miriam's attention. She was innocent of any plan or act of murder, but nonetheless, because it was related to her, "the suspicion of being at least an accomplice to the crime fell darkly and directly" (p. 431) on her. Miriam avows to Kenyon, "But you know that I am innocent" (p. 431). She was exonerated but what became a widely-publicized scandal enveloped her and prompted her flight to Rome where she adopted the pseudonym of Miriam Schaefer. When the Model reminds her of "the power that I have over you" (p. 96), he alludes to his ability to publicly reveal her true name which was a watchword of the scandal; this leverage constitutes the "later thraldom" in which he holds her. He preys on Miriam's fear that she will be shunned by her new community of friends, perhaps as had happened in the aftermath of the murder. Miriam, under mounting strain and with "an insatiable instinct that demands friendship, love and intimate communion" (p. 114) has a peremptory need for the support of her friends and fears being alienated from them. And it proves to be true after she reveals her name to Kenyon, the sculptor immediately identifies the horrific event and reacts viscerally to it.[15] In *The Scarlet Letter*, Chillingworth holds Hester in a similar thrall regarding the public revelation of Dimmesdale as her partner in adultery.

The provocation for this murder, hidden in plain view, can be constructed retrospectively by what transpires between Donatello and the Model. The Model is intolerant of Donatello's attentions to Miriam, as he intrudes on them at every turn in the road. Given the prominent place in *The Marble Faun* for what Freud will later call the repetition compulsion, "that terrible event," I conjecture, was the result of the violence between the Model and a man who had been captivated by Miriam's beauty and, like Donatello, was a rival for her company and affection. Sensing with great fear that a calamity is about to be repeated, Miriam tries, unsuccessfully, to warn off both men. She gives the reader a clue as to the nature of the murder in her rebuke of Donatello when she becomes aware that he observes her in a silent fit of rage in the shadows of the Colosseum: "How dare you look at me? …Men have been struck dead for a less offence!" (p. 157). I believe she did not mean this assertion metaphorically but as a history.

It is almost certainly the Model who stuck the fatal blow at an offender, as he bears the psychic burdens of a man who has committed a murder. Once again presuming to touch Miriam without invitation, the Model takes Miriam's hand and inspects it "as if to discover some imaginary blood-stain" and comments, "I have known hands…which all the waters of the ocean could not have washed clean" (p. 97). The hands he knows in this way are his own, as Miriam's retort regarding her hand makes clear: "It had no stain until you grasped it with your own" (p. 97). The Model enacts his statement's image when he washes his hands at the Trevi Fountain: "Dipping his hands into the capacious wash-bowl, the Model rubbed them together with the utmost vehemence" (p. 147). Like Lady Macbeth's, all great Neptune's ocean cannot wash the blood clean from a murderer's hand.

The characterization of the crime as "mysterious" may help account for the fact that the Model had somehow eluded civil authority, but he could not escape punishment by his outraged superego. His guilt "led him to a convent, where his severe and self-inflicted penances had even acquired him the reputation of unusual sanctity" (p. 432). The sadism in his treatment of Miriam is turned against himself in the masochistic gratification afforded him in his life in the Capucin brotherhood.[16] Like Dimmesdale in *The Scarlet Letter*, the Model is caught in an unresolvable conflict between desire and conscience, and, as Chillingworth accurately diagnoses in his patient, is prey to: "all the fear, the remorse, the agony, the ineffectual repentance, the backward rush of sinful thoughts, expelled in vain!" (Hawthorne, 1962, Vol. 1, p. 139). The Model had struggled successfully to stay away from Miriam, but their encounter in the Catacomb, "destroyed the work of years" (p. 96). As with an addict who relapses when he takes the first drink, pill, or fix, his addiction to Miriam is rekindled with undiminished force. The work of guilt repeats itself as Donatello's conscience sets him on the path blazed by the Model: first, painful withdrawal from Miriam and then, masochistic self-abnegation, intermixed with compulsive ritual religious practice.[17]

Like Hilda, who is stained by only observing a murder, so Miriam is all the more stained by a murder committed because of her. Innocence of the act does not spare either of the young women from the truth that "[e]very crime destroys more Edens than our own!" (p. 212). In her own estimation, Miriam has become a femme fatale. She enjoins her young admirer: "If you were wiser, Donatello, you would think me a dangerous person….if you follow my footsteps, they will lead you to no good" (p. 80). The erotic attention the Model paid her when she was a child, made Miriam feel herself the source of powerful and destructive attraction; the murder the Model committed because of her reinforced this conviction. She exclaims to Donatello: "They call me beautiful; and I used to fancy that, at my need, I could bring the whole world to my feet" (p. 158).

Miriam's Sketches: The Power of Women

With abundant artistic talent, intelligence and generosity of spirit, Miriam establishes herself in Rome and, out from under the dark shadows of the Model and the scandal involving him, she can exult that she has "escaped from all the past!" (p. 96) and "had made for [herself] a new sphere, and found new friends, new occupations, new hopes and enjoyments" (p. 96). Her friendships, in particular, had "given her almost her first experience of happiness" (p. 431). However, her traumatic past overtakes her in "that ill-omened adventure of the catacomb" (p. 432).[18]

Miriam is once again tormented by the man who "blasted her sweet childhood." Perhaps in a repetition of how she was manipulated by him as a child, the Model threatens to expose her if she does not yield to him. After he sets forth these conditions in the Borghese Grove, she becomes increasingly desperate. Significantly, however, she also reacts with anger at his oppression: "I hate him, too!" she tells Donatello after the Model interrupts their sylvan dance. The depth of the anger, and fantasies of murderous revenge associated with it, find expression in Miriam's portraits of Jael, Judith, and Salome, committing acts of violence against men. Miriam can disguise the deeply personal content of these portraits because she is working within the well-established medieval and Renaissance artistic *topos*, "the power of women," in which are depicted scenes, often Biblical, in which strong men who are dominated by women.[19] Maryan W. Ainsworth and Joshua P. Waterman (2013) write that this genre presents "an admonitory and often humorous inversion of the male-dominated hierarchy" (p. 59). However, there is nothing humorous about the destructive urge that underlies Miriam's pictures of a man being murdered by a woman. It represents Miriam's wishes to turn passive victimhood into commanding aggression and exact revenge on her tormentor. She is accurate in her self-awareness that, as she tells Donatello, "they are ugly phantoms that stole out of my mind; not things that I created, but things that haunt me" (Hawthorne, 1962, Vol. 2, p. 45). These fantasies will be translated into reality when they steal out of her haunted mind as the Model's life hangs in the balance on the edge of the Tarpeian Rock.

Kenyon's Cleopatra

Agitated by the confrontation with the Model and the ultimatum he just delivered, Miriam visits Kenyon's studio in distress. As a woman alone and threatened, she needs to unburden herself of her secret plight and receive a friend's sympathy. Later in her visit she tells Kenyon: "There is a secret in my heart that burns me!...Ah, if I could but whisper it to only one human soul" (p. 128).[20] Kenyon's sculpture of Cleopatra sways Miriam to consider him as the person that she will take into her confidence.

As a subject of his new work, the sculptor chooses a queen of fabled beauty at the moment when she is contemplating a momentous confrontation. The narrator remarks, "The expression was of profound, gloomy, heavily revolving thought; a glance into her past life and present emergencies, while her spirit gathered itself up for some new struggle or was getting sternly reconciled to impending doom" (pp. 126–127). As I believe was true of Hilda's portrait of Beatrice Cenci, Kenyon, moved by a sensitive attunement to Miriam, is capturing in the stone figure of Cleopatra what he has apprehended to be his friend's urgent mental state.[21] Indeed, Miriam, at that very moment, stands on the precariously narrow ground between her troubled past and an ominous future.[22]

"Cleopatra" is also a tribute to the allure that Kenyon finds in Miriam's physical beauty. The narrator notes the "softness and tenderness" in the form which is, at the same time, "fierce, voluptuous, passionate, tender, wicked, terrible and full of rapturous enchantment" (p. 127). Miriam, it would seem, has awakened more of *Eros* than Kenyon can comfortably handle, and he resists the wish to yield himself to her as "conquered territory" (p. 48). Another sculpture that he shows to Miriam of a pearl-fisher fatally entangled in weeds at the bottom of the sea (p. 117) expresses his fear of the dangers of sexual arousal. His infatuation with the idealized Dove, Hilda, is far less of a threat.[23]

Seeing her woman's dilemma so accurately represented in "Cleopatra," Miriam is tempted to divulge her secret to its sculptor. Kenyon hesitates and, though no word is spoken, withdraws slightly his receptivity to the intimacy. Miriam, exquisitely sensitive, accurately reads his reluctance: "Miriam looked into his eye, and detected it at once" (p. 129). Kenyon recovers from this momentary lapse and is prepared to be engaged, but it is too late for Miriam, who departs shortly thereafter and finds "her Shadow waiting for her in the street" (p. 130).

All is determined in what is read in a fleeting glance, as will be true at the Tarpeian Rock. Hawthorne instructs us that every moment counts: the brief empathic misalignment between friends may have vast implications. If Miriam had been able to relieve her troubled psyche to Kenyon, she might have been spared calamity. In the scene on the Campagna, she confesses to Kenyon her urge to reveal her story: "On one occasion, especially, (it was after you had shown me your Cleopatra,) it seemed to leap out of my heart, and go as far as my very lips. But, finding you cold to accept my confidence, I thrust it back again. Had I obeyed my first impulse, all would have turned out differently" (p. 433).

Toward the Precipice

With fear and rage stifled, Miriam endures the lighthearted mood of the aesthetic company during the midnight ramble in and around Rome's historic sites. The Model stalks her at each turn of the way, while Miriam's and Donatello's agitation rise. At the Trevi Fountain, in an action which indicates a loosening of control over aggression, Miriam flings water "into her persecutor's face" (p. 147). Donatello is sufficiently inflamed to have "seized violently" (p. 148) Miriam's arm and he assures her that if "[you] bid me to drown him...You shall hear his death-gurgle in an instant!" (p. 148). Donatello is signaling to Miriam that he is prepared to act as an extension of her will. Miriam, consciously wanting no violence, attempts to calm him down: "Peace, peace, Donatello!"...Do him no mischief!...What it is to you or me, Donatello? There, there! Be quiet, foolish boy!" (p. 148).[24] As the Model pursues her into the shadows of the Colosseum, Miriam's distress finds expression in a wordless tantrum in which she "began to gesticulate extravagantly, gnashing her teeth, flinging her arms wildly abroad, stamping her feet" (p. 157). Miriam is approaching the breaking point. Sensing an imminent crisis and fearing a repetition of "that terrible event," she pleads with Donatello to "flee from me...there is a great evil hanging over me... it will crush you, too, if you stand at my side...Cast me off; or you are lost forever!" (p. 158). Donatello will not be dissuaded and he proclaims: "I will never quit you" and, with this pledge of devotion, he wins Miriam's confidence, if not yet her love (p. 158). She is moved to affirm: "And I will accept his aid! Tomorrow—tomorrow—I will tell him all" (p. 158). Miriam has come to value the seriousness of Donatello's offering very differently from earlier when "He held out his love so freely, in his open palm, that she felt it could be nothing but a toy" (p. 80).

Tomorrow, as it turns out, is too late. At the Piazza del Campidoglio, Miriam is drawn to the imposing equestrian statue of Marcus Aurelius, about which she fantasizes: "Oh, if there were but one such man as this...Then, how speedily would the strife, wickedness, and sorrow of us poor creatures be relieved! We would come to him with our griefs...even a poor frail woman, burthened with her heavy heart—and lay them at his feet, and never need to take them up again. The rightful King would see to all!" (p. 166). In this re-enactment of a scene from long ago, Miriam is expressing the urgent longing, unmet in her childhood, for a father who can see her victimhood and will protect her from the abuser.

Thoughts of death are in the air as the company arrives at the parapet overlooking the Tarpeian Rock. Miriam considers suicide as a way to escape her crisis: "It would be a fatal fall, still!...Even without the weight of a burthened heart, a human body would fall heavily enough upon those stones to shake all its joints asunder. How soon it would be over!" (p. 169). The discussion of the fate of traitors of the Roman republic who were thrown to their death at that very site, affords Miriam the chance to express retaliatory fantasies against the Model under the guise of historical commentary. To Donatello's question as to who the men were who were punished in this manner, Miriam answers, "Men whose lives were the bane of their fellow-creatures. Men who poisoned the air, which is the common breath of all, for their own selfish purposes. There was short work for such men, in old Roman times" (p. 170). Donatello then asks: "Was it well done?" In a reply that is replete with meaning, Miriam replies: "It was well done...Innocent persons were saved by the destruction of a guilty one, who deserved his doom" (p. 170).

Thus all is primed for the denouement. Miriam's warnings to Donatello and the Model have not been heeded. She harbors volcanic emotions and Donatello has also been aroused to the point of violence; he has taken assurance that punishment of a villain is just. Human nature takes its course. As we find out later from Hilda's account of the scene, the Model emerges from a niche and approaches Miriam who falls to her knees in front of him. Donatello, undoubtedly outraged by this posture of servility, seizes the Model and holds him over the precipice. Miriam must see her predator in this vulnerable pose before her psyche shuts down. In that brief but momentous interval, murderous wishes that have gathered for years toward her persecutor press for gratification; these are simultaneously countered by the superego's prohibition against murder. The magnitude of the anxiety associated with conflict floods her psyche and results in a dissociated mental state. Although her consciousness is clouded, the text that is writ large in the unconscious cannot be obscured: the wish to see the Model destroyed can be read in her eyes, both by Donatello and Hilda. "I did what your eyes bade me do, when I asked them with mine, as I held the wretch over the precipice!" (p. 172), Donatello tells her. Hilda elaborates on the content of the look in her eyes: "It revealed all your heart, Miriam! A look of hatred, triumph, vengeance, and, as it were, joy at some unhoped for relief!" (p. 210). With the constraints of consciousness lifted, the ghosts in Miriam's haunted mind are released and Hilda has identified them correctly. Sublimation was possible by painting canvases representing the power of women, but is not available to Miriam in the wild reality of the scene. The Model is thrown to his death without a word and Miriam's tragic fate is sealed. Miriam's earlier musing, stimulated by viewing Kenyon's sculptures, take on added relevance here: "As these busts in the blocks of marble, so does our individual fate exist in the limestone of Time. We fancy that we carve it out; but its ultimate shape is prior to all our actions" (p. 116). Carton (1992) astutely comments that "Freud's and Hawthorne's narratives both convey a feeling that may be described as a strange combination of the sense of fatality and the sense of chaos" (p. 100).

Poor Criminals

Throughout the inexorable progression to the denouement, the narrator has built a sympathetic case for Miriam's plight as an admirable and accomplished woman who has been tormented in childhood and as an adult by a man who also has the blood of violent crime on his hands. Despite Miriam's rational arguments, impassioned entreaties and warnings, the Model persists in his pernicious design to possess or destroy her. In his disdain for Roman governance, the narrator makes it clear that, as in the time of Beatrice Cenci, no appeal to Papal authority will bring this man to justice. Moreover, the narrator repeatedly conjures the Model in ways that offend the moral sense of the reader: he is likened to the "Spectre of the Catacomb" who betrayed the saints and refused an opportunity for salvation (p. 40); he is referred to as the "Shadow" (p. 130), a "Man-Demon" (p. 33), a "sinister personage" (p. 92), and his face, according to Hilda, resembles that of the Devil in Guido's drawing of the triumph of the Archangel Michael. Kenyon imagines him as a Roman conqueror dragging a captive Miriam in public humiliation through the streets of Rome.

It is breath-taking, then, how the narrator, having built his case against the Model, immediately turns on Miriam and judges her a criminal. Although she falls into a lapsed state of consciousness and never utters a word of assent to Donatello, she is nonetheless condemned by the narrator as "the guilty, blood-stained, lonely woman" who, when she recovers clarity of mind, turns to "her fellow-criminal...whom she had drawn into her doom" (p. 173). The narrator has just practiced what he conjectured had been Miriam's artistic touch in her drawing of Jael slaying Sisera: "Miriam had added a certain wayward quirk of her pencil, which at once converted the heroine into a vulgar murderess" (p. 43). This moral bait-and-switch reveals a facet of the quixotic nature of the narratorial voice. Hawthorne, through this unanticipated "wayward quirk" in the narrator's perspective, has flung the reader into a moral labyrinth around the enigma that Miriam ponders in Guido's Beatrice: "I would give my life to know whether she thought herself innocent, or the one great criminal since time began!" (p. 67).

Miriam comments earlier in the narrative: "But what a strange efficacy is in Death!" (p. 117). Indeed, with the Model's death, Miriam's life is changed forever. At the moment of her release from a long subjection to the Model, she is inextricably bound to the consequences of a violent act against him that set her free. Like Beatrice Cenci, punishment of her tormentor exacts a very high price. Unlike Beatrice, however, in the very midst of this act, Miriam finds love. The bond to the Model had crowded out her psychic landscape and created a barrier to human intimacy. With Donatello's valorous action against her enemy, "the voiceless gulf" (p. 113) between herself and others is bridged; she had called out, "Help, friends, help!" (p. 113) and Donatello had heard her. He had made good on his pledge: "If you desire it, or need it...I shall not be loth to die!" (p. 157). In performing this act, Donatello has helped heal a wound inflicted by childhood trauma. As in a fairy tale, when the courageous hero has vanquished the enemy, he wins the beautiful heroine's heart; after long tribulations, Miriam has been readied to enter the enchantment of romance. Love for Donatello and concern for his welfare will consume her from then on. In their interchange in the Marble Saloon, Miriam tells Kenyon "If Donatello is entitled to aught on earth, it is my complete self-sacrifice" (p. 283). The narrator's reflections on the profound impact of Donatello's intervention explain a great deal about the heroine's psychology: "But in Miriam's eyes, Donatello was always, thenceforth, invested with the tragic dignity of their hour of crime; and furthermore, the keen and deep insight, with which her love endowed her, enabled her to know him far better than he could be known by ordinary observation. Beyond all question, since she loved him so, there was a force in Donatello worthy of her respect and love" (p. 284). The dignity and tragedy of the love born during the hour of their crime evolves in the remainder of *The Marble Faun.*

Miriam and Donatello

Donatello and Miriam need time to integrate the aftershocks of the Model's death and their roles in it. For Miriam, there is immediate relief from the isolation that the bondage to the Model had imposed upon her. She proclaims: "only yesterday, only a half-hour ago, I shivered in an icy solitude... No friendship, no sisterhood, could come near enough to keep the warmth within my heart. In an instant, all is changed! There can be no more loneliness!" (p. 175). Donatello is now for her, "my one, own friend!" (p. 173). Miriam wants Donatello to share her excited sense of liberation: "Forget it! Cast it all behind you!...The deed has done its office, and has no existence any more" (p. 176). In this she succeeds, but the narrator makes it clear that the freedom from the superego and the guilt it wields, will be brief: "They flung the past behind them, as she counselled, or else distilled from it a fiery intoxication through those first moments of their doom. For guilt has its moments of rapture, too. The foremost result of a broken law is ever an ecstatic sense of freedom" (176).[25] Even in the midst of excitement, Miriam senses the brevity of relief as she exclaims, "To-night, at least, there shall be no remorse!" (p. 177). The narrator, assuming the voice of punitive conscience, insists on being heard through the veil of fleeting bliss that surrounds the couple, as he speaks of: "the ever-increasing loathsomeness of a union that consists of guilt. Cemented with blood, which would corrupt and grow more noisome forever and forever, but bind them none the less strictly for that!" (p. 175).

Their elation is indeed brief as it has dissipated by the time Miriam and Donatello meet in the morning for the planned rendezvous with Kenyon and Hilda at the Church of the Cappuccini: "How icy cold is the heart, when the fervour, the wild ecstasy of passion, has faded away, and sunk down among the dead ashes of the fire that blazed so fiercely" (p. 178).[26] Miriam finds ample strength to encounter the Model in the unexpected form of the dead Capucin. She confronts the sternness of his look and defiantly addresses his corpse: "No, thou shalt not scowl me down! Neither now, nor when we stand together at the Judgment Seat. I fear not to meet you there" (p. 191). Her words recall Beatrice's challenge to her father: "Frown not on me! Haste, hide thyself, lest the avenging looks of my brothers' ghosts should hunt thee from thy seat!" (Shelley, p. 29, lines 151–153). Miriam has confidence in her case against the Model that she will argue before the ultimate Judge. I believe that neither she nor Beatrice have guilt or remorse over the murders, per se; in the judgment of each, the perpetrator got the justice he deserved. Miriam insists to Kenyon: "It is not remorse! Do not think it! I put myself out of the question and feel neither regret nor penitence on my own behalf" (p. 280). The source of remorse and penitence for Miriam will lie elsewhere.

However, Donatello's conscience is unforgiving: "My heart shivers... Nothing, nothing will ever comfort me!" (pp. 196–197). Guilt over the murder of the Model begins to afflict him despite Miriam's fervent avowal: "Let me bear all its weight. I am well able to bear it; for I am a woman, and I love you! I love you, Donatello. And surely you love me?" (p. 198). Donatello murmurs his answer, "I did" as he withdraws his hand from hers. In that gesture, Miriam realizes that the love she has long sought, and that glowed so intensely the day before, has become remote, if not completely lost. She now considers it a "sad mistake" to have hoped Donatello held a love for her "vital enough to survive the frenzy of that terrible moment; mighty enough to make its own law, and justify itself against natural remorse" (p. 199).[27] With her sophisticated mind and independent spirit, Miriam might have been capable of attempting to transmute an act of murder into something other than a crime through "a love, annihilating moral distinctions" (p. 199). Donatello, despite the force and sincerity of his love, does not have that capacity. He is left with the burden of guilt for having violated what for him is a sacred law. Realizing that her presence is disruptive to Donatello, as it brings "in its train, the remorse and anguish that would darken all your life," Miriam bids him "Leave me, therefore, and forget me!" (p. 200). She offers a promise that expresses nobility and generosity of purpose: "But if ever –in distress, peril, shame, poverty, or whatever anguish is most poignant, whatever burthen heaviest –you should require a life given wholly, only to make your own a little easier, then summon me!... May you never need me more! But if otherwise, a wish—almost an unuttered wish—will bring me to you!" (p. 200). Miriam will be true to this vow. Donatello's act of love is reciprocated by her dedication to palliate his suffering in any way at her command.

Once Hilda confirms what Donatello saw in her eyes, Miriam unambiguously embraces her part in communicating an assent to the act of murder: "I accept my own misery...my own guilt, if guilt it be, and whether guilt or misery, I shall know how to deal with it" (p. 197). That she was not fully conscious and cannot remember the scene, does not mitigate her sense of responsibility for Donatello's action. Miriam is a woman of magisterial integrity. Early in the narrative she worries about Donatello's attachment to her: "Ah, what a sin, to stain his joyous nature with the blackness of a woe like mine!" (p. 158); after the murder, she reproaches herself for not having been more forceful in repudiating his attention to her: "Why did I not drive you from me, knowing –for my heart foreboded it—that the cloud, in which I walked, would likewise envelope you!" (p. 197). Having failed to do so, she must "seek to remedy the evil you have incurred for my sake!" (p. 198). Her misery and guilt originate in a sense of the destructiveness of her physical beauty and are a part of the legacy of the incestuous relationship to which the Model had subjected her. Long before Hilda, Miriam was marked in childhood to be "'Innocence, dying of a Blood-stain'" (p. 330). If Miriam can be said to have a tragic flaw, it is her fatal beauty. As her self-portrait reveals, she is all too aware of the power it exerts. Her acceptance of her lot is noble in its selflessness: "As for myself, I am past mine own or others' pity" (p. 199). Within a day of Miriam's being freed from her nemesis, Hilda rejects her and Donatello withdraws to Monte Beni with Kenyon soon to follow, making a bitter irony of what she had exclaimed the night before: "There can be no more loneliness!" (p. 175).

Miriam becomes a Shadow who follows Donatello to Monte Beni. Her song, which inspires the hope of redemption, signals to him that she is there; she is distraught that he does not respond to its call. Miriam's love for Donatello requires her presence if he needs her, as he is "The object, which I am bound to consider my only one on earth" (p. 280). However, her woman's heart has opened and the love that resides there leaves her startlingly vulnerable. To be worthy of Donatello's love has become her *raison d'être*: "With this object before me I feel a right to live! Without it, it is a shame for me to have lived so long!" (p. 283).[28]

Kenyon may have lacked requisite sympathy earlier, but he manifests an abundance of it in the crucial brotherly role of protector and counselor. He admirably fulfills the duty of friendship and is of considerable help to Donatello at Monte Beni. After close observation of him in his distraught state, Kenyon concludes that Donatello still loves Miriam, but, because of what the sculptor considers his misguided urge for self-punishment, he will not allow himself the love and succor she could offer. Kenyon reassures Miriam: "...he not only loves you still, but with a force and depth proportionate to the stronger grasp of his faculties, in their new development" (p. 282). This affirmation of Donatello's love, after all, has a powerful transformative effect on Miriam and is described in the most refulgent passage in the romance: "'But, he loves me...Yes; he loves me!' It was strange to observe the womanly softness that came over her, as she admitted that comfort into her bosom. The cold, unnatural indifference of her manner, a kind of frozen passionateness, which had shocked and chilled the sculptor, disappeared. She blushed and turned away her eyes, knowing there was more surprise and joy in their dewy glances than any man save one ought to detect there" (p. 282).[29]

David B. Kesterson (1973) convincingly finds parallels between Kenyon and Donatello's wanderings from Monte Beni to Perugia and Virgil and Dante's spiritual journey from Purgatorio to Paradiso. Both seekers, Dante and Donatello, are spiritually prepared by their sojourn for a redemptive union with a beatific woman. Thus there are resonances between Miriam and yet another famous Beatrice. At the journey's end and at the appointed spot under the statue of Pope Julius II, Donatello calls out for Miriam and, as admits to her: "...my deepest heart has need of you" (p. 320). Donatello simple words tell Miriam all that she has longed to hear: "first of all, he still loved her. The sense of their mutual crime had stunned, but not destroyed the vitality of his affection; it was therefore indestructible" (p. 319). Moreover a penitent Donatello asks her forgiveness: "Forgive, Miriam, the coldness, the hardness, with which I parted from you. I was bewildered with strange horrour and gloom" (p. 320).

Although reunited, but still under a shadow of the murder, Miriam and Donatello are perplexed as to how to proceed and seek Kenyon's guidance. Through the months of attending to Donatello and from his interchanges with Miriam, Kenyon has arrived at a profound understanding of what befell his friends: "when I think of the original cause, the motives and feelings, the sudden concurrence of circumstances thrusting them onward, the urgency of the moment, and the sublime unselfishness of either part—I know not well how to distinguish it from much that the world calls heroism" (p. 384). Kenyon relies on an epistemology grounded in sympathy. He then expresses, in the form of a paradox, the romance's central moral question: "Might we not render some such verdict as this? –Worthy of Death, but not unworthy of Love!" (p. 384). All that we have gathered about Miriam and her life story supports an affirmative answer to his question. I believe that Hawthorne chooses Kenyon as the spokesperson for the wisdom that is closest to his own mind and heart and, in doing so, undercuts the narrator's stern and conventional judgments. [30] Although it eluded him in his studio, Kenyon here gives Miriam "just the kind of sympathy…that the occasion required" (p. 129).

The sculptor, in a sage reckoning, exhorts Miriam and Donatello to share the burden of their calamity through a soulful union of mutual support, self-sacrifice, and good works. They can never hope to live in the fantasy that "The deed has done its office, and has no existence any more" (p. 176); instead, they must find a way to live within the compass of its hard reality. The couple accepts both the austerity and rightness of Kenyon's prescription, whose authority does not seem to derive from an identifiable religious teaching, but is certainly Christian in its aspiration toward a higher life. Miriam and Donatello's union may take place under the beneficent gaze of the bronze statue of the Pontiff, but the priestly blessing over them is recited by Kenyon: "The bond betwixt you, therefore, is a true one, and never, except by Heaven's own act—should be rent asunder" (p. 321). Miriam will reciprocate and sanctify Kenyon and Hilda's union at the romance's conclusion.

After the severity of their trials, the couple is offered a unique dispensation, and the narrator adds an optimistic note regarding it: "Who can tell where happiness may come…Perhaps–shy, subtle thing–it had crept into this sad marriage-bond" (p. 323). And in an exuberant Dantean vision, the narrator observer that Donatello "held Miriam's hand; and there they stood, the beautiful man, the beautiful woman united forever" (p. 323). However, Kenyon has added a proviso to their union which haunts their brief wedded life: "If ever, in your lives, the highest duty should require from either of you, the sacrifice of the other, meet the occasion without shrinking!" (pp. 322–323). When the time arises that the stipulation needs to be enforced, a Divine Comedy is transfigured into Human Tragedy.

For Hilda and Kenyon

Millington (1992) forcefully argues that there are two distinct narrative voices in *The Marble Faun*, one for Miriam, which arises from her complexity and one for Hilda which speaks for her innocence. Each voice "produces a chorus of mutually antagonistic moral pronouncements, observations, witticisms, and explanations" (Millington, 1992, p. 195). In this interesting but extreme view, *The Marble Faun* "is the disorienting form of narrative civil war" (p. 196) in which what he views as Hilda's narrative triumph signals "the defeat of romance" (p. 181). Although I concur that the narrative voice is complex, a psychological reading finds more points of intersection and sympathy between Miriam and Hilda than the image of civil war will allow. They were, after all, the closest of friends, who cared deeply about each other until the Model's death created a chasm between them.[31] Miriam's love for Hilda bridges the divide.

Miriam, concerned that Hilda is alone and despondent in Rome, urges Kenyon to return from Perugia to be her companion, and he promptly heeds her direction. His reunion with Hilda in St. Peter's and her abduction soon after, occupy the next several chapters of the novel. Miriam and Donatello, now in a position to live out a renewed life together, disappear from the foreground of the narrative. The time of their unfettered union is brief. Miriam, the reader later learns, has connections with powerful authorities in Rome, and through these she must early on be made aware of Hilda's abduction and its relation to the secret she divulged in the confessional.[32]

Thus, it is a time of moral crisis for the recently joined couple. Hilda had been a friend to whom Miriam had professed: "If I deemed it good for your peace of mind…to bear testimony against me, for this deed, in the face of the world, no consideration of myself would weigh with me an instant" (p. 211). Loyal friendship, both toward Hilda and Kenyon, necessitates that she and Donatello bear witness against themselves in exchange for Hilda's freedom. The Dove is, after all, innocent and they are not. The reader recalls that after the murder, Miriam urgently pleads with Hilda: "Then be more my friend than ever, for I need you more!" Despite Hilda's repudiation of her, when it is her turn, Miriam heeds friendship's urgent call. All too soon, Miriam and Donatello reach the juncture, in accord with Kenyon's stipulation, that their highest duty demands the sacrifice of the other.

The reader is not told about their deliberations. It is clear that Miriam has no faith in Roman justice and perhaps had hoped to arrange Hilda's release some other way. However, she yields to Donatello's determination that his case must be brought before the proper authorities of the Papal state. For better or worse, as part of his transformation, the Faun has developed a mind of his own. The arrangement is made *sub rosa*: Hilda will be released at the instant that Donatello and Miriam are arrested. Kenyon knows nothing of it at the time, and Hilda perhaps never learns what was done to gain her release.[33] This secret is also kept from the reader, but Miriam, while always maintaining her dignity, betrays the terrible pain of the immanent separation from the man she loves.

When Kenyon presses her about Hilda's release, Miriam replies: "I should like to play round this matter, a little while, and cover it with fanciful thoughts, as we strew a grave with flowers. But I linger and hesitate, because every word I speak brings me nearer to a crisis from which I shrink" (p. 428).[34] Miriam begs her partner for more time: "Ah, Donatello, let us live a little longer the life of these last few days! It is so bright, so airy, so childlike, so without past or future" (p. 428). Donatello grants another precious day. The narrator has prepared the reader for the pathos of Miriam's plea by his reflections on the enormity of the history of Rome against which "our own life is nothing" (p. 410), and yet, he opines, the "heart cries out obstreperously for its small share of earthly happiness…How wonderful, that this our narrow foothold of the Present should hold its own so constantly, and, while every moment changing, should still be like a rock betwixt the encountering tides of the long Past, and the infinite To-come!" (p. 411). Miriam has cried out and, as a consequence, she and Donatello stand together for one more day on the rock of the Present.

When we reflect on it, the parting of friends is exquisitely poignant. Unaware of what is about to unfold, Kenyon attempts to hurry the reunion with Hilda and Miriam again rebukes him: "You are yourself unkind to come between us at this hour. There may be a sacred hour, even in Carnival-time!" (p. 448). There is a consecration to Miriam and Donatello's last moments together. In her comments on the Fall of Man, Miriam imparts to Kenyon her insights on the potential of sin, and the toil and sorrow it brings, to prompt the spirit to attain "a higher, brighter and profounder happiness" (p. 434). The pain of impending loss, however, overshadows these uplifting reflections. Kenyon discerns the "profound sadness in her tone, overpowering its momentary irritation, and assuring him that a pale, tear-stained face was hidden behind her mask" (p. 448). After holding hands in a circle, the friends part from each other with a final "Farewell!" (p. 448). At that terrible moment, we recall the narrator's earlier somber counsel: "For it is thus, that, with only an inconsiderable change, the gladdest of objects and existences become the saddest; Hope fading into Disappointment; Joy darkening into Grief, and festal splendour into funereal duskiness" (p. 226).

In the Preface to *The Cenci*, Shelley states that "The highest moral purposes aimed at in this highest species of drama, is the teaching of the human heart, through its sympathies and antipathies, the knowledge of itself; in proportion to the possession of which knowledge, every human being is wise, just, sincere, tolerant and kind" (p. 4). Shelley and Hawthorne were kindred spirits. Through trauma and suffering, and mediated by love, Miriam acquires profoundly sad and uplifting knowledge of the human heart and is transformed by it into a woman who can be treasured as wise, just, sincere, tolerant and kind. It is fitting at the end that we recall the judgment: "Worthy of Death, but not unworthy of Love!"

Aftermath

Under the Eye of the Pantheon, in direct communication with the Deity, Kenyon and Hilda are betrothed in gladness, hope, joy, and the expectation, when they return home, to be celebrated in festal splendor. Miriam, saint-like in a penitent's garb, silently blesses their union as she "stood on the other side of a fathomless abyss, and warned them from its verge" (p. 461).[35] Like Hester Prynne, Miriam has become a woman in mourning and "burdened with a life-long sorrow" (Hawthorne, 1962, Vol. 1, p. 263); and, as was befitting the tragic heroine of *The Scarlet Letter*, we can foresee for Miriam a spiritual path upon which similarly she will spend "toilsome, thoughtful and self-devoted years" (Vol. 1, p. 263) that will make up the rest of her life.

Although Miriam removes herself from Kenyon and Hilda, as well as the reader, she will be remembered. As a wedding gift, she bestows upon Hilda her bracelet, which was "composed of ancient Etruscan gems, dug out of seven sepulcres, and each one of them the signet of some princely personage, who had lived an immemorial time ago" (Hawthorne, 1962, Vol. 4, p. 462). The bracelet reminds Hilda of a "fanciful legend of the adventures and catastrophe of its former wearer" that Miriam composed. It is the memory of Miriam's art as a storyteller that brings Hilda, finally, to tears. Hawthorne ends *The Marble Faun* not with the defeat of romance, but by asserting its unique power to effect and transform.

The memory of her friendship with Miriam, and all it involved, will find its place in the depth of Hilda' art. The Dove returns as a married woman to the familiar terrain of New England and with Kenyon as a devoted and artistically inspired partner. In this setting, there is every reason to believe that as an artist she will fulfill the potential that the narrator finds in her: "With years and experience, she might be expected to attain a darker and more forcible touch, which would impart to her designs the relief they needed" (p. 55). And it is Hilda that Hawthorne invests with the exalted vision which, we can imagine, served to inspire writing *The Marble Faun*: "Would not this be an admirable idea for a mystic story, or parable, or seven-branched allegory, full of poetry, art, philosophy, and religion! It shall be called 'The Recovery of the Sacred Candlestick'. As each branch is lighted, it shall have a differently colored lustre from the other six; and when all the seven are kindled, their radiance shall combine into the intense white light of Truth!" (p. 371).

Notes

1. Kenyon is aware of Hilda's emotional limitation and alludes to the capacity that she will need to develop: "she is abundantly capable of sympathy, and delights to receive it, but she has no need of love!" (p. 121).
2. Evan Carton (1992) points out that the term "haunted" appears more than fifty times in the novel (p. 51).
3. Hilda's full statement to Kenyon is as follows: "Nobody, I think, ought to read poetry, or look at pictures or statues, who cannot find a great deal more in them than the poet or artist actually expressed. Their highest merit is suggestiveness" (379).

4. One does not need to be a psychoanalyst to suspect that Miriam serves as a displacement for Crews's never-directly articulated hostility toward Hawthorne.
5. For the record, Miriam did not have Donatello kill the Model.
6. Will and Mimosa Stephenson. Oxymoron in *The Marble Faun. Nathaniel Hawthorne Review* 21 (1995) 1-13. The number of oxymorons in the text is not specified in the essay; Mimosa Stephenson estimated the number as four hundred and fifty in a personal communication (2018).
7. Mathé (1992) draws on Rimmon-Kenan's (1971) study of ambiguity whose conclusions are relevant to a discussion of *The Marble Faun*: "the creation of ambiguous works is one of art's ways of solving the problem of contradictories–solving it not by choice but by an artistic dramatization of their coexistence" (Rimmon-Kenan, 1971, p. 234).
8. The prosody of Dimmesdale's Election Day sermon in *The Scarlet Letter* strikes similar cords: "At times this deep strain of pathos was all that could be heard, and scarcely heard, sighing amid a desolate silence" (I:243).
9. David Greven (2012) discusses Hawthorne's experience of being mesmerized by the extraordinary beauty of the Jewess, Emma Abigail Montefiore Solomons, wife of the Lord Mayor of London, who was sat across from him at a dinner that he attended while U.S. Consul in Liverpool. Hawthorne was captivated by her "Jewish" beauty and his descriptions bear a strong resemblance to the compelling quality of narrator's attraction to Miriam's self-portrait. Greven's essay elaborates on the complex topic of Miriam's purported Jewishness and its bearing on her relationship to the Model, amongst other things.
10. Whatever allegorical or unconscious meaning one might want to assign to the encounter in the Catacomb, the narrator provides sufficient context so that their meeting can find a place as a chance encounter in the realm of a realistic novel. The Model, who has entered the brotherhood of the Capuchin order in Rome, was visiting the Catacomb in search of penance in its holy confines for the murder he committed. Miriam has no prior knowledge of this identity as a monk nor his whereabouts. For the four friends, the Catacomb was one of the many popular tourist sites that they made a practice of visiting together. It is part of the Model's egotistical frame of mind, one which hints at insanity, that he asserts "[she] came to me when I sought her not. She called me forth, and must abide the consequences of my reappearance in the world" (Hawthorne, 1962, Vol. 4, p. 31). Miriam did not seek him, and given her abhorrence for this man, it is clear that it was he who could not let go of her after the chance meeting. Miriam reminds him: "you might have suffered me to glide past you like a ghost, when we met among those shadows of ancient days. Even now, you might bid me pass as freely" (p. 96).
11. "The Model," the title to which this character is generally referred, is an ironic moniker based on the group of artists' observation of his frequent visits to Miriam's studio. Certainly his appearances in her studio were unwanted intrusions; although Miriam indeed made many sketches of him, perhaps in an effort to exorcise his demonic influence, he was certainly not functioning as her "model". Perhaps it would be iconoclastic, but not otherwise lacking in merit, to refer to him throughout by his name, Brother Antonio. Similarly, "Donatello" and "the Dove" were nicknames assigned to the Count of Monte Beni and Hilda respectively. Of course, "Miriam Schaefer" (p. 39) is a pseudonym.

12. In *The Scarlet Letter*, Chillingworth and Hester are also of disproportionate ages; however, despite her later bitter regret, Hester entered the union willingly.
13. Brenda Wineapple (2003) reports that Hawthorne had read the play in the mid-1840's. While in England, he visited with Leigh Hunt, to whom *The Cenci* was dedicated. (See entry Leigh Hunt, poetryfoundation.org). Shelley's famous work was on Hawthorne's mind as he was preparing to write *The Marble Faun.*
14. Leonard Shengold's (1989) description of soul murder is applicable to important aspects of the Model's treatment of Miriam: "Soul murder is neither a diagnosis nor a condition. It is a dramatic term for criminal behavior, the deliberate attempt to eradicate or compromise the identity of another. The victims of soul murder remain in large part possessed by another, their soul is in bondage to someone else. The capacity to destroy a soul hinges entirely on having another person in one's power and the helplessly dependent is inherent in childhood" (p. 19).
15. Nathalia Wright (1943) connects "that terrible event" with the murder of the Duchesse de Praslin by her husband, a crime which gained international attention in the press. Henriette Deluzy-Desportes, who had served as the Praslin governess, was investigated as to her possible role in inciting the murder; she was eventually exonerated. The specific details of this murder are not relevant for the story of *The Marble Faun*: Miriam is not Mlle. Deluzy. Hawthorne invokes a crime of passion of this sort as an example of the disrepute that stains anyone, however innocent, who is associated with it. Miriam was trying to escape ignominy by establishing herself in Rome. We think in our own time of the power of the names linked to such highly publicized crimes as Charles Manson's murder of Sharon Tate or the abduction of Patty Hearst. It is not at all clear that, despite her fears, Miriam's closest friends would have rejected her if they discovered her identity. Miriam's fear of this prevents her from putting her friends to the test. Difficulty establishing trust is another consequence of childhood trauma.
16. The hated Model, of whom Miriam says, "there was nothing viler during his lifetime," (p. 191) had a side that was unknown to Miriam. He had gained a reputation for sanctity as a monk and undoubtedly performed good works that brought women and children to the Church of the Capuccini to mourn his death. Miriam reacts to his humanity when, naïve to his religious calling, she intimates that he might find solace in prayer. At this suggestion: "He looked so fearfully at her, and with such intense pain struggling in his eyes, that Miriam felt pity" (p. 96).
17. Dimmesdale's unconfessed guilt enforces a separation between Hester and himself and likewise results in self-punishing religious ritual. The Reverend's psychological deterioration is detailed in Chapter Two.
18. In *The Blithedale Romance*, Zenobia establishes a new foundation for her life in the Blithedale community until her past overtakes her in the persons of Priscilla, Old Moodie, and Westervelt. Zenobia's relationship to her past is explored in Chapter Four.
19. See Susan Louise Smith's (1995) *The Power of Women: A Topos of Medival Art and Literature.*
20. In *The Scarlet Letter*, Dimmesdale also has had an intense need to divulge his secret, as he tells Hester: "Thou little knowest what a relief it is, after the torment of a seven years' cheat, to look into an eye that recognizes me for what I am!" (Vol. 1, p. 192).

21. Carton (1992) finds evidence for the same conclusion: "Hawthorne intimates that Miriam herself may have been the model for 'the womanhood' that Kenyon has embodied in Cleopatra" (p. 72).
22. As with Hilda's Beatrice as well as Miriam's self-portrait and sketches of the women doing violence, Kenyon's Cleopatra is another instance of the unique capacity of an artwork to mediate the virtually inexpressible workings of the human spirit. The narrator admits that it was Kenyon's final unfinished bust of Donatello, in which he "sees propounded...the riddle of the Soul's growth, taking its first impulse amid remorse and pain, and struggling through the incrustations of the senses" (Vol. 4, p. 381), that interested him in the man's history and which ultimately impelled him to write *The Marble Faun*.
23. It is good to remember that Kenyon was enamored with Hilda long before Miriam appeared on the scene in Rome. However, his attraction to Miriam endures. In the Marble Saloon he admits to her, "May I tell you, Miriam... that you are still as beautiful as ever?" (p. 286).
24. Nor is this the first time that Miriam had to quell Donatello's impulsivity which he wants to channel in the service of protecting her. When the Model interrupts their dance in the Borghese Gardens, Donatello gives his rival "a look of animal rage" and mutters, "I hate him!" to which Miriam, in the first intimation of a conspiracy, responds, "Be satisfied; I hate him, too!" Taking license form this exclamation, Donatello queries, "Shall I clutch him by the throat! Bid me so; and we are rid of him forever!" Miriam restrains him, "In Heaven's name, no violence!" (p. 91).
25. Hester's exhortation to Dimmesdale in *The Scarlet Letter* is in the same vein, and, in the end, equally unsuccessful: "Leave this wreck and ruin here where it hath happened! Meddle no more with it! Begin all anew!" (Vol. 1, p. 198).
26. This passage suggests that Miriam and Donatello consummated a sexual union the previous night.
27. In *The Scarlet Letter*, Hester anticipates Miriam's attempt to define a law of her own. In the face of her years of punishment by the community, the narrator concludes that for Hester, "The world's law was no law for her mind!" (Vol. 1, p. 164). In the forest scene, she reminds Dimmesdale that, regarding their sexual union, "What we did had a consecration of its own. We felt it so! We said so to each other!" (p. 195).
28. While in Rome, Margaret Fuller, who had been a close friend of Hawthorne at one time, married Giovanni Osoli, a man who was pure in his affection and intensely devoted to her, although far below her intellectual accomplishment. Much to her friends' surprise, Fuller, who had eschewed marriage, reciprocated his love and developed a strong emotional dependence on him. Although Hawthorne voiced skepticism about the union, there are elements of it in his rendering of Miriam's unanticipated love for Donatello. See Megan Marshall's (2014) excellent biography, *Margaret Fuller: A New American Life*.
29. The effect of the reaffirmation of love on Miriam is reminiscent of that of Hester's renewed love with Dimmesdale: "There played around her mouth, and beamed out of her eyes, a radiant and tender smile, that seemed gushing from the very heart of womanhood. A crimson flush was glowing on her cheek, that had long been pale" (Vol. 1, p. 202).
30. David Greven's (2018) insightful comments on this passage suggested this conclusion.

31. While it is true that Hilda's rejection of Miriam is unfeeling and extraordinarily hurtful, she does eventually realize her failing as a friend: "'Miriam loved me well', thought Hilda, remorsefully, "and I failed her at her sorest need!'" (p. 386). Moreover, it is in keeping her promise and delivering Miriam's packet to the Palazzo Cenci, that she is abducted. One need remember, too, that Hilda knew nothing of Miriam's history of abuse at the hands of the Model; such knowledge might have mitigated her uncompromising judgment of her friend's role in the murder.
32. It is apparent that the priest who heard Hilda's confession must have reported its content to the authorities. It was he who sits on the balcony with an English family at Carnival and gives Kenyon a gesture of recognition at the moment Hilda is released into their midst.
33. In response to Hilda's perplexity as how her release was obtained, the narrator coyly suggests, "We can only account for it by supposing that the fitful and fantastic imagination of a Woman…had arranged this incident, and made it the condition of a step which her conscience, or the conscience of another, required her to take" (p. 456). Although both are arrested, Donatello is sent to prison but Miriam is ultimately released. In the Postscript, Hawthorne interjects a central irony in Kenyon's explanation to Hilda of Miriam's presence in the Pantheon "Call it cruelty, if you like—not mercy!... But, after all, her crime lay merely in a glance; she did no murder" (p. 467).
34. The grave they are strewing is Donatello's. Having sent to his death a member in good standing of the Capucin order, Roman justice undoubtedly would call for Donatello's execution or, at very least, life imprisonment. Arnold Goldman (1984) sets the novel's action precisely between April 1858 and March 1859 (p. 383). It was a time of marked political turmoil in Rome. After the collapse of the Roman republic in 1849, which was established as part of the larger effort to unify Italy against Papal authority, there were strenuous efforts by the Papacy to suppress and punish any manifestations of civil disorder. The French gendarmes which are omnipresent in the narrative were enlisted by the Pope to that end (Kolish, 2001, p. 438).
35. Several critics see this betrothal as regressive not progressive. For Baym (1971), Kenyon's fear of losing Hilda again compels him into "lying like a frightened child to placate her" and thereby win her acceptance. In a widely over-reaching conclusion, Baym judges that his fear demonstrates that he is "ludicrously inadequate for the vocation he had so bravely chosen for himself" (p. 374). Millington (1992) is also severe in his assessment of this union: "The sculptor seeks protection from his own complexity of mind and erects Hilda as an icon of moral simplicity, a charm against ambivalence. Hilda's acceptance takes the form of an acknowledgement of her own need for protection, her permanent childhood" (p. 186). Miriam would hardly do well to offer a benediction for such a betrothal. It is important to remember that Kenyon arrived at the guiding wisdom for Miriam and Donatello; it is unlikely, having come that far, he will renounce moral complexity and ambivalence. Like Holgrave at the conclusion of *The House of the Seven Gables,* a young man can make accommodations for his dearly beloved without compromising his integrity. As for Hilda, it is part of her psychological development to move beyond a self-sufficiency which is inimical to intimacy; the experience of vulnerability and a need for protection are prerequisites for mature love. Kenyon and Hilda are just beginning their journey together.

References

Ainsworth, M., & Waterman, J. (2013). *German Paintings in the Metropolitan Museum of Art, 1350–1600*. New York: The Metropolitan Museum of Art.

Arvin, N. (1961). *Hawthorne*. New York: Russell and Russell.

Baym, N. (1971). *The Marble Faun*: Hawthorne's Elegy for Art. *The New England Quarterly, 44*.

Carton, E. (1992). *The Marble Faun: Hawthorne's Transformations*. New York: Twayne Publishers.

Chodorow, N. J. (1999). *The Power of Feelings*. New Haven: Princeton.

Crews, F. (1996). *The Sins of the Father: Hawthorne's Psychological Themes*. New York: Oxford University Press.

Dunne, M. (2004). Tearing the Web Apart: Resisting Monological Interpretations *in The Marble Faun*. *South Atlantic Review, 69*.

Goldman, A. (1984). The Plot of Hawthorne's The Marble Faun. *Journal of American Studies, 18*.

Gollin, R. (1975). Painting and Character. *ESQ, 21*.

Greenwald, E. (1991). Hawthorne and Judaism: Otherness and Identity in *The Marble Faun*. *Studies in the Novel, 23*.

Greven, D. (2012). Hawthorne and the Gender of Jewishness: Anti-Semitism, Aesthetics, and Sexual Politics in *The Marble Faun*. *The Journal of American Culture, 35*, 35.

Greven, D. (2018). Personal Communication.

Hall, S. (1970). Beatrice Cenci: Symbol and Vision in *The Marble Faun*. *Twentieth Century Fiction, 25*.

Hawthorne, N. (1962a). *The Blithedale Romance*. In W. Charvat (Ed.), *The Centenary Edition of the Works of Nathaniel Hawthorne* (Vol. 3). Columbus: Ohio State University Press.

Hawthorne, N. (1962b). *The House of the Seven Gables*. In W. Charvat (Ed.), *The Centenary Edition of the Works of Nathaniel Hawthorne* (Vol. 2). Columbus: Ohio University State Press.

Hawthorne, N. (1962c). *The Marble Faun*. In W. Charvat (Ed.), *The Centenary Edition of the Works of Nathaniel Hawthorne* (Vol. 4). Columbus: Ohio State University Press.

Hawthorne, N. (1962d). *The Scarlet Letter*. In W. Charvat (Ed.), *The Centenary Edition of the Works of Nathaniel Hawthorne* (Vol. 1). Columbus: Ohio State University Press.

Hunt, L. (n.d.) Retrieved from The Poetry Foundation: poetryfoundation.org

Hutner, G. (1988). *Secrets and Sympathy: Forms of Disclosure in Hawthorne's Novels*. Athens, Georgia: University of Georgia Press.

Kesterson, D. (1973). Journey to Perugia: Dantean Parallels in *The Marble Faun*. *ESQ, 19*, 94–104.

Kolish, A. (2001). Miriam and the Conversion of the Jews in Nathaniel Hawthorne's *The Marble Faun*. *Studies in the Novel, 33*.

Marshall, M. (2014). *Margaret Fuller: A New American Life*. New York: Houghton Mifflin.

Mathé, S. (1992). The Reader May Not Choose: Oxymoron as Central Figure of Hawthorne's Strategy of Immunity from Choice in *The Scarlet Letter*. *Style, 26*(4).

Millington, R. H. (1992). *Practicing Romance: Narrative Form and Cultural Engagement in Hawthorne's Fiction*. Princeton: Princeton University Press.
Rimmon-Kenan, S. (1977). *The Concept of Ambiguity–the Example of James*. Chicago: University of Chicago Press.
Shengold, L. (1989). *Soul Murder*. New Haven: Yale University Press.
Shelley, P. B. (1886). *The Cenci: A Tragedy in Five Acts*. London: Reeves and Turner.
Smith, S. (1995). *The Power of Women: A Topos of Medieval Art and Literature*. University of Pennsylvania Press.
Stephenson, W., & Stephenson, M. (1995). Oxymoron in the Marble Faun. *Nathaniel Hawthorne Review*, *21*, 1–13.
Ullén, M. (2004). *The Half-Vanished Structure: Hawthorne's Allegorical Dialectics*. Bern: Peter Lang.
Von Abele, R. (1955). *The Death of the Artist: A Study of Hawthorne's Disintegration*. The Hague: Marinus Nijhoff.
Wineapple, B. (2003). *Hawthorne: A Life*. New York: Knopf.
Wright, N. (1943). Hawthorne and the Praslin Murder. *The New England Quarterly*, *15*, 5–14.

6 Hester's Return to Boston in *The Scarlet Letter*: "Her whole orb of life both before and after, was connected with this spot, as with the one point that gave it unity"

The Problematic Conclusion

In the Conclusion of *The Scarlet Letter*, "many years" (Hawthorne, 1962, Vol. 1, p. 261) after her departure from New England with Pearl, Hester Prynne returns alone to reside in her former cottage in Boston and "of her own free will" (p. 263) resumes wearing the scarlet letter until the end of her long life. Pearl, who is to marry and resettle abroad in an "unknown region" (p. 262) would have "joyfully entertained her sad and lonely mother at her fireside" (p. 262). At a crossroads, Hester chooses instead to return to New England where "there was more real life for her" (p. 262). In a succinct statement of her motivation for this action, the narrator states: "Here had been her sin; here her sorrow; and here was yet to be her penitence" (p. 263). And so it was to be.

Sacvan Bercovitch (1988) underscores the interpretive dilemma posed by the Conclusion: *The Scarlet Letter*'s "most problematic aspect [is] the dramatic moment when Hester decides to come home to America....This particular drama has gone unappreciated, no doubt because it is absent from the novel. At a certain missing point in the narrative, through an unrecorded process of introspection, Hester Prynne abandons the high, sustained self-reliance by which we had come to identify her...[and] chooses for no clear reason to abandon her heroic independence, and acquiesces to the A after all. She returns voluntarily to the colony that had tried to make her 'a life-long bond-slave'" (p. 631). Hester's fate is generally considered, in the contemporary critical imagination, as indeed problematic, if not frankly incendiary: having won the reader's admiration for "her heroic independence" and having suffered mightily under the burden of the scarlet letter imposed by the Puritan magistrates, why would she choose to return, "for no clear reason," to the site of her torment and willingly replace on her breast the hated token of her shame and oppression? The Hester we have come to respect and admire would not, it would seem, have made such decision "of her own free will." Many critics concur that it goes against the grain; something is wrong here.

Sandra Tomc (2002) summarizes "the overwhelming sense among twentieth-century critics...is that Hawthorne demonstrates a kind of lapse in these pages, and that whether Hester's return evinces an ideological seam or simply a glaring aesthetic mistake, some crucial energy in the novel has been suppressed, coerced, disciplined, thwarted, silenced or disallowed" (p. 490). In this formulation, Hester, of course, is the source of the crucial energy that vivifies *The Scarlet Letter* and Hawthorne, her creator, is the agent of her oppression. Nina Tassi (1998) gives voice to the refrain of critical sentiment that "it is the author who brings his heroine back. Why, except out of a desire to punish her does he return her to that dreary place forever" (p. 34). There are many speculations as to what motivates the author's impulse to punish. Tassi, for one, hypothesizes it involves a conflict over sexuality: "...perhaps he is punishing himself for having let her burst forth in the forest to forbidden sexual mastery over a lover only too much like himself" (p. 34). Harold Bloom (2004) relates Hester's final subjugation to Hawthorne's status as an artist: "[Hester] fails her art, which may be the cost of Hawthorne's not failing his, and it may be that Hester's compromised condition at the book's close is the consequence of being sacrificed by the author as a substitute judgment for himself" (p. 4). Larry J. Reynolds (1988) suggests that Hawthorne is settling a personal score: "More than one reader has correctly surmised that this ending of the novel constitutes a veiled compliment to Hawthorne's little Dove, Sophia, and a veiled criticism of Margaret Fuller –radical, advocate of women's rights and subject of gossip because of her child and questionable marriage" (p. 79). Michael J. Colacurcio (1972) stresses that Hester "reaches certain antinomian conclusions" but, in the end, "the tale and the teller force her to abandon those conclusions" (p. 480). Gillian Brown (1991) believes that Hester's return as "a domestic angel" is Hawthorne's "capitulation of nineteenth-century conventional ideal of womanhood" (p. 34). Nina Baym (1970), more charitably, sees that Hester's return "is meant to symbolize the limits of a woman's freedom, circumscribed by love" (p. 222).

Whatever the author's putative motivation, and there are many other theories about it, Tassi (1998) feels that "Hawthorne has no mercy for Hester" (p. 34) and as a most unfortunate consequence, Robert Stanton (1970) avers, her admirable spirit is broken: "her change springs from exhaustion and defeat not inspiration; she has lost her feelings, she has lost her sensitivity to the Puritan's cruelty and hypocrisy; she has lost hope. Her one source of happiness, Pearl's marriage, is dropped into the story like a winning lottery ticket" (p. 28). Frederick I. Carpenter's (1988) pronouncement is blunt: "In his 'Conclusion' therefore, Hawthorne did violence to the living character whom he had created"(p. 68). Interpretations of this kind would lead one to conclude that Hester fared far better under seven years of Puritan authority than under authorial tyranny which consigned her to the life-long position as his own bond-slave. We need to be clear about the nature of these critics' accusations: if Hester's return to Boston is not, as stated in the text, an exertion "of her own free will" but the forceful imposition of an authorial will inimical to hers, Hawthorne has committed, according to his own moral hierarchy, an unpardonable sin. As with fiendish Chillingworth in relation to

Dimmesdale, the author "has violated, in cold blood, the sanctity of a human heart" (p. 195).

It is a formidable irony of literary history that a book considered among the most, if not *the* most influential work of fiction in the American literary canon (Buell, 2014), finds its Conclusion widely judged, 'a glaring aesthetic mistake' and, at worst, sustained violence against a nation's most beloved fictional heroine. The irony is compounded because such a failure would betray the rigorous aesthetic credo that Hawthorne (1962) espouses in the Preface to *The House of the Seven Gables* regarding the artistic integrity of a novel, from start to finish: "A high truth, indeed, fairly, finely, and skillfully wrought out, brightening at every step, and crowning the final development of a work of fiction, may add an artistic glory, but is never any truer, and seldom more evident, at the last page than at the first" (Vol. 2, pp. 3–4). But what, we may ask, if the "last page" is less true by far than the first or frankly false, and its crowning final development is an egregious aesthetic mistake? Or, no better, if "the darkening close of a tale of human frailty and sorrow" (p. 48), as it is anticipated by the narrator at the end of the romance's first chapter, constitutes an awkwardly seamed, unintegrated, ideological appendage? Henry James, who wrote the first comprehensive assessment of Hawthorne's oeuvre, espouses an exacting standard for a novel's aesthetic integrity akin to Hawthorne's: "in proportion as the work is successful the idea penetrates it, informs and animates it, so that every word and every punctuation contribute to the expression" (Sganlon, 1962, p. 214).[1] Apparently James, attuned to every word and punctuation, was insensible to the artistic failure of *The Scarlet Letter*'s ending as it is not mentioned in his commentary which, instead, expresses highest admiration for the novel's literary virtue: "It is beautiful, admirable, extraordinary; it has in the highest degree of that merit which I have spoken of as the mark of Hawthorne's best things – an indefinable purity and lightness of conception" (James p. 57).

This study accords with James' estimation. In this pre-eminently psychological novel which inscribes the characters' entangled and tormented conflicts with, in F.O. Matthiessen's (1941) phrase, "psychological exactitude" (p. 277), a psychoanalyst finds himself very much on familiar ground. And as a clinician who in the consulting room makes a practice of attunement to what Nancy J. Chodorow (1999) refers to as psychoanalysis's distinctive provenance, "the power of feelings," I find the Conclusion of *The Scarlet Letter* adheres to the truth of Hester's human heart, yes, in every word and punctuation. This study proffers a counterpoint to the strain of contemporary critical judgment that takes exception, and in such pejorative terms, to the romance's Conclusion which, I must confess, always brings me to tears. In it, I feel, Hester is elevated, not debased, and that it is indeed the romance's crowning development. I draw on textual precedent for taking the unusual step to advance my feelings as evidence in a scholarly paper: in The Custom-House introduction, the narrator's encounter with the old scarlet letter communicated "some deep meaning in it, most worthy of interpretation, and which, as it were streamed forth from the mystic symbol subtly communicating itself to my sensibilities, but evading the analysis of my mind" (Vol. 1, p. 31). I am not alone in falling under the spell that *The Scarlet Letter* casts over its reader. In an 1850 review written shortly after the novel's publication, Anne Abbott describes what she calls the "magic power" of Hawthorne's style: "when [the reader] closes the book, he will feel very much like the giddy and bewildered patient who is just awakening from his first experiment of the effects of sulphuric ether. The soul has been floating or flying between earth and heaven, with dim ideas of pain and pleasure strangely mingled, and all things earthly swimming dizzily and dreamily, yet most beautiful, before the half shut eye" (Abbott, 1988, p. 31). More recently, Sylvie Mathé (1992) tersely echoes Abbott's experience: "*The Scarlet Letter* vibrates with wonder" (p. 626).[2] So, too, throughout almost two centuries of innumerable readers' encounters with *The Scarlet Letter*, does it communicate its truths powerfully and directly to the sensibilities. Unbiased by ever-shifting ideological trends in critical analysis, the romance's readers exemplify Hawthorne's insight that "the uninstructed multitude...forms its judgment...on the intuitions of its great and warm heart, the conclusions thus attained are often so profound and so unerring, as to possess the character of truths supernaturally revealed" (Vol. 1, p. 127). And our great and warm hearts, I will argue, are drawn most prodigiously toward Hester Prynne because of her ultimate fate, not despite it.

Ernest Sandeen (1962) accurately judges that Hawthorne "has directed the bias of our sympathy toward Hester....Hester is the empathic center" (p. 435). This chapter is a cross-discipline study of the romance's "empathic center" in which I will apply a psychoanalytic lens to the text in order to elucidate the motivations, conscious and unconscious, which bring Hester back to Boston. Chodorow (1999) contrasts psychoanalytic epistemology with that of other humanistic disciplines in that it is "first and foremost an account and theory of personal meaning;" psychoanalytic technique is employed toward interpreting that meaning by "unraveling the particularistic uniqueness of each individual psyche and history" (p. 129). As Hawthorne knew and Freud was to confirm from the analysis of neurotics, the past is recorded in the unconscious and forever exerts its influence on the present. Thus, the entirety of Hester's past is encoded in her return to Boston. Accordingly, I will use what we come to know and can reasonably infer about Hester's life and character in order to construct a psychoanalytically informed narrative which serves as the foundation for interpreting the psychological dynamics of her momentous return to the Bay Colony. Hawthorne's rendering of Hester's psychology is complex and the narrative which seeks to unpack it, is, of necessity, lengthy. However, "the power of feelings" will serve, to use Mathé's (1992) felicitous phrase, "like Ariadne's thread through the treacherous maze of the tale" (p. 607).

To anticipate my findings: there is abundant evidence that the Conclusion has been thoroughly foreshadowed in the text and that it is integral to it. Hester's return to Boston, after long years abroad, is indeed an expression of her own free will: it is a heroic effort at a critical juncture of her life, when the parental responsibility of raising Pearl is complete, to re-work into usable forms the traumas she suffered as the wearer of the scarlet letter. Chief among these is the death of her beloved, Arthur Dimmesdale: as an extended act of mourning, she identifies with him as a guide to a path of redemption. The Conclusion witnesses Hester, with enduring determination, transforming her tormented past into a life of sustained social value and spiritual beauty. Having earlier been the object of scorn, she gains from the community the "reverence due to an angel" (p. 32). Based on her experience of painful isolation, she returns to be a resource of support, wisdom, and spiritual inspiration for women in similar distress. That she is drawn back to Boston, and to the scaffold which was the site of shame, guilt, and death, exemplifies the power of the unconscious forces which inheres in Freud's concept of the return of the repressed: "her whole orb of life, both before and after, was connected with this spot, as with the one point that gave it unity" (p. 244). Hester returns to Boston to bring her life to unity—psychologically, morally, and spiritually.

The Narrative Gap

Before proceeding with Hester's narrative, it is important to focus on a crucial narrative gap which significantly influences any attempts to interpret the heroine's motivations. Bercovitch (1988) points out that Hester's decision to return to Boston takes place "at a certain missing point in the narrative, through an unrecorded process of introspection." Indeed it does; in fact, that "missing point" falls somewhere toward the end of a subtly executed but nonetheless stunning narrative gap regarding Hester which begins abruptly after her final interchange with Dimmesdale on the scaffold and spans some two decades until her reappearance at the threshold of her former dwelling.[3] The reader loses track of Hester at the moment the minister dies. Although the narrator records the reactions of others who witness his scene on the scaffold, he utters not a word about Hester's, whose prolonged suffering and anticipation of release in an imminent departure with the minister and Pearl have engaged the reader's deep sentiments. In but a few fateful minutes Hester has lost, forever, the man she "once…and still so passionately loved" (Vol. 1, p. 193), with whom she recently shared the fantasy that soon he would be walking "hand in hand with us" and, together they would have "a home and fireside of our own" (p. 212). The only mention of her, chilling in its abstractness, and even then not by name, is in relation to Chillingworth's death a year later: "But, in no long time after the physician's death, the wearer of the scarlet letter disappeared, and Pearl along with her" (p. 261). Hester disappears from the reader stealthily and in the manner that she does from Boston a year later—quietly, without notice.

But what of the inner life of Hester Prynne to which we have hitherto been intimate participants from the moment of her dramatic appearance on the scaffold of shame? What did she experience in Dimmesdale's unanticipated confession of guilt and long-delayed acknowledgment of her as his partner and Pearl as his daughter? What of their now thwarted departure, toward which "the whole seven years of outlaw and ignominy had been little other than a preparation" (p. 200)? What of mother and daughter after Pearl's transformative kiss and, above all, what of the profound encounter, in the attitude of a *Pietà*, with her lover's death in her arms? As if she received a traumatic blow to the head, Hester is stunned into silence. Moreover, having been a victim of dehumanizing public exposure on that very scaffold and for the years after as the wearer of the scarlet letter, with this narrative gap, I propose, Hester is shielded by Hawthorne from the reader's gaze; he has secured her "inmost Me behind its veil," (p. 4) a veil of silence. At this time of trauma and utmost vulnerability, there will be no repetition of a voyeuristic violation of the sanctity of Hester's human heart.

Hawthorne further disorients the reader by collapsing years of time into a few paragraphs of text. This textual time warp is a two-decade hiatus from Hester's participation in the scene of the minister's death until the veil is finally lifted. Thus it is not only the "process of introspection" surrounding "the dramatic moment" in which Bercovitch imagines Hester makes a decision to return to Boston that is absent from the narrative, but *all* of her internal processes go unrecorded from the moment of Dimmesdale's death until the narrator breaks the silence in the Conclusion: "But there was more real life for Hester Prynne, here, in New England, than in that unknown region where Pearl had found a home. Here has been her sin; here, her sorrow; and here was yet to be her penitence. She returned, therefore, and resumed, –of her own free will…the symbol of which we have related so dark a tale" (pp. 262–263). Hester, some twenty years later, at last, is brought back to narrative life.

As significant as the scene of Dimmesdale's death is to Hester, the narrative gap raises many other questions. How did Dimmesdale's revelation influence the community's view of Hester and Hester's relation to the community? That she "disappears and Pearl with her," with no goodbyes to anyone, suggests a persistent alienation, on her part, at least. That Chillingworth deteriorates and dies about a year after Dimmesdale's death, but not before he bequeaths a substantial fortune to Pearl, suggests a repentance as his death approached. In any case, Pearl departs "the richest heiress of her day, in the New World" (p. 261) and settles with Hester in the Old World, presumably in England where she can be raised and educated free of Puritan restraints. Now with abundant wealth at their disposal, we can imagine that their life is significantly different from the one they were forced to live as outcasts in a little cottage by the sea. What transformations were effected in Hester's psyche during twenty years of a life of social privilege in the intellectual and religious freedom afforded by her more progressive homeland? What became of the convictions of the woman who, at one time, had been "alone, and hopeless of retrieving her position" (p. 164) when she undoubtedly could attain, if she desired it, a significant social standing and whose daughter's status allows her entrée into marriage with an aristocrat? Although she had, one time "cast away the fragments of a broken chain," was it still true, years later, that "The world's law was no law for her mind" (p. 164)? Or might it be that, like Holgrave's radicalism in *The House of the Seven Gables,* so too for Hester, "when, with the years settling down more weightily upon him his early faith should be modified, it would be by no harsh and sudden revolution of sentiments" (Vol. 2, p.180)? The narrative gap prevents the reader from finding explicit textual answers to these questions, which, I hope to show, can be sought in the narrative of the remainder of Hester's life in Boston.

Bercovitch is correct that "the silence surrounding Hester's conversion to the scarlet letter is deliberate on Hawthorne's part by forcing us to represent it for ourselves, by ourselves" (p. 650)[4]; this chapter is just such an attempt to represent it psychoanalytically. In his own interpretive effort, Bercovitch locates what he considers the critical moment in the text when Hester's fate is cast. This occurs as she impatiently awaits the end of the Election procession which stands between her and the departure with Dimmesdale and Pearl. At that anxious moment she feels extreme alienation from the crowd which is gathered about her. She fantasizes addressing them: "Look your last on the scarlet letter and its wearer!... Yet a little while and she shall be beyond your reach! " (p. 227). Bercovitch then asserts, with a certitude that is remarkable, "That is why Hawthorne must bring her back. It is as though under pressure of her resistance the letter were slipping out of his control, losing its efficacy as an agent of reconciliation" (p. 650). Bercovitch has concluded that Hester is somehow assigned by Hawthorne to be that agent of reconciliation and thus, as a moral requisite, she must fulfill "the office of the scarlet letter." Hawthorne through Hester urges the social imperative that, in Bercovitch's words, "we may subject ourselves through self-expression to the cultural premise of ambiguity" (p. 652). And he concludes: "This is what Hester learns during her unrecorded period of self-scrutiny in the old world" so that she can be "voluntarily, an exemplar of continuity through integration" (p. 636). Thus Bercovitch's interpretation, taking as its point of reference Hester's state of mind before Dimmesdale's final ascent on the scaffold, excludes any consideration of all that Hester experiences in the narrative gap. Most glaring, in this regard, is the failure to take into account the profound impact on Hester of Dimmesdale's death and its aftermath. As we shall see, the scene of the minister's death exerts a singularly compelling influence on Hester's return to Boston. In addition, his interpretation does not consider changes inevitably wrought by time in her long residence as woman of means in England. It is as though Bercovitch suspends Hester in a frozen state at a moment of vengeful and rebellious thoughts against the community, then thaws her out in the Old World long enough for her to see her "antinomian" impulses for what they were and thereby enable a "conversion to the scarlet letter" which allows her to accept the author's philosophy of social integration. In Bercovitch's imaginings, Hester leads no real life in the interim. With reference to *The Scarlet Letter,* R.W.B. Lewis (1955) writes, "narrative deals with experiences not propositions" (p. 3). Although influential for a generation of critics, Bercovitch's interpretation of Hester's return to Boston is seriously, if not fatally flawed in its failure to consider the possibilities of all that transpires and is transformed during the narrative gap, one which he has taken pains to bring to readers' attention.

Hester Prynne, Before the Fall

Whenever possible, a psychoanalytic inquiry begins with childhood during which, as Freud was to systematically explicate, psychic structures are formed which are the foundation for the development of adult character. Although we are told relatively little of Hester's childhood, we know that it is the groundwork for her gem-like character which, as Tassi extols, "a century and a half after her creation… continues to bedazzle her readers" (p. 23).

Hester, "the child of honorable parents" (p. 79), was a young woman who enjoyed a "happy infancy and stainless maidenhood" (p. 80) in a home in England which had a "poverty stricken aspect, but retaining a half-obliterated shield of arms over the portal in token of antique gentility" (p. 53).[5] As a defense against mental anguish on the scaffold, Hester enters into a dissociative state in which she conjures loving images of her parents during childhood. Her father's face is imagined "with its bald brow, and reverend white beard, that flowed over the old-fashioned Elizabethan ruff" (p. 58). Her mother's image is recalled with its "look of heedful and anxious love," the memory of which had so often, even after her death, served as "a gentle remonstrance in her...pathway" (p. 58). Her mother's watchful concern had been internalized and came to her assistance by serving as an impediment to what we later learn is her "impulsive and passionate nature" (p. 57). As fate will have it, this aspect of her nature is the locus of what might rightly be called, in terms of the romance's tragic cast, Hester's tragic flaw.

Her next association on the scaffold, as if he were *in loco parentis*, is to Chillingworth, the significantly older and physically deformed scholar who courted her. One can speculate that Hester's mother was already deceased at the time of this courtship, for under her "heedful" surveillance, his suit might not have been successful. As with Zenobia in *The Blithedale Romance* and Miriam in *The Marble Faun,* things may go terribly awry in a young woman's love life without the benefit of maternal guidance. Be that as it may, Chilllingworth was a man of significant scholarly accomplishment and, as the reader finds out much later, of substantial wealth. His own estimation of his character is confirmed by Hester: "thoughtful of others...kind, true, just and of constant, if not warm affections" (p. 172). Undoubtedly, he sought to overcome his life-long isolation and find comfort in the warm glow of Hester's youth. It is never stated, but altogether possible, that Chillingworth's pursuit of a union with a young and beautiful woman served as compensation for the damage done to his self-image by his congenital deformity. This would help explain the severity of the injury done to him by Hester's adultery and his implacable need for revenge against the virile man who had possessed her. Chillingworth confesses: "I drew thee into my heart, into its innermost chamber, and sought to warm thee by the warmth which thy presence made there!" (p. 74). We can see everything that is wrong emotionally for Hester in Chilllingworth's formulation of their relationship as he offers no warmth of his own, only that which has already emanated from her. Nonetheless, she married him and in the interview in prison she concedes,"I have greatly wronged thee" (p. 74).[6] Seven years later she becomes aware, in horror, that, as manifest in his torture of the minister, her husband has been transformed from an honorable man into a fiend. At that realization, "The scarlet letter burned on Hester Prynne's breast...Here was another ruin, the responsibility of which came partly home to her" (p. 170). For Hester, it was not the act of adultery alone which is the source of guilt, but the "bane and ruin" that it brought to both her husband and lover that eventually brings her to seek repentance.

Chillingworth, not without insight of his own, later admits to her that he "betrayed thy budding youth into a false and unnatural relation with my decay" (p. 75). Hester was young and inexperienced: "in the time when her heart knew no better," he had persuaded her to "fancy herself happy by his side" (p. 176). In promoting this fantasy Chillingworth had "imposed on her" (p. 177) a "marble image of happiness" (p. 177) instead of its "warm reality" (p. 177). Hester knew enough of her own feelings to admit to him at the time that she did not love him: "thou knowest that I was frank with thee. I felt no love; nor feigned any" (p. 74). In retrospect "[s]he marvelled how she could ever have been wrought upon to marry him!" (p. 176). The words "betrayed," "imposed" and "persuaded" all qualifying Chillingworth's influence on Hester, shed light on the ways he manipulated her, inexperienced as she was, to accept his hand in marriage. We see how Chillingworth again exerts his influence over a vulnerable Hester through forceful persuasion as he exacts an oath of silence from her in the prison cell.

Chillingworth's violation of Hester's innocence provokes her fall. Daniel Cottom (1982) considers the unnatural union in marriage of Chillingworth to Hester as "the original sin from which arises the sin of adultery" (p. 55). Much later, after her confrontation with Chillingworth, Hester comes to a similar conclusion, although in very different terms: "She deemed it her crime most to be repented of, that she had ever endured and reciprocated, the lukewarm grasp of his hand, and had suffered the smile of her lips and eyes to mingle and melt into his own" (Vol. 1, p. 176). Hester admits to herself that in this charade of affection toward Chillingworth, she had committed a "crime" against her own nature by misrepresenting the true promptings of her heart. The narrator clearly judges that Chillingworth did an injustice to Hester as well as to himself by winning her hand but not "the utmost passion of her heart" (p. 176). Instead, in a marriage likely never consummated, (Ellis, 1980, p. 55)[7] and with an aging and physically unattractive man, Hester had to content herself with the "lukewarm grasp of his hand" (p. 176). Such tepidity was not sufficient to incite Hester's latent sexuality.

For this she was to wait for another man, with "some mightier touch... to awaken...all her sensibilities" (p. 176). This man was to be her Reverend, Arthur Dimmesdale.

Hester lived alone for well over a year awaiting Chillingworth to join her in the Bay Colony. Nothing had been heard from him since his departure from Amsterdam and there was a general presumption that he was no longer alive. Thus she bore the susceptibility of a woman alone and precariously situated in a new and not necessarily hospitable community. Chillingworth alludes to having followed, at some time, the Puritan doctrine, but the reader does not know with any precision the nature or depth of Hester's religious commitment. Undoubtedly, "as the daughter of a pious home" (p. 111), Hester had been raised in the Christian faith and her embrace of Puritan tenets must have satisfied the Boston Elders' rigorous interrogation, a requisite in that time and place, for anyone being granted admission to the church community.[8]

Hester's relationship with Dimmesdale was *ab initio* that of parishioner to pastor. When Reverend Wilson addresses her on the scaffold, he refers to Dimmesdale as "my young brother, here, under whose preaching of the word you have been privileged to sit" (p. 65). In the Governor's Hall, she appeals to Dimmesdale to prevent Pearl from being taken from her and she reminds him of their prior formal relationship, although she is also making subtle allusion to their personal liaison: "Thou wast my pastor, and hadst charge of my soul, and knowest me better than these men can" (p. 113). Alone as she was, there is no reason to believe that, as her minister, Dimmesdale did not take steps to be of assistance to her and that he did not excel in his office toward her as he did for the entire community. From various sources in the text it is possible to collate a portrait of Dimmesdale, before the sexual fall with its disastrous emotional consequences, that shows him to be a young man of extraordinary character and accomplishment: he was an Oxford graduate of "scholar-like attainments," "high native gifts" and "eloquence and religious fervor" (p. 66); he was, in essence, a "young and eminently distinguished divine" (p. 238) who had come to the New World as Puritan minister to bring "all the learning of the age into our wild forest-land" (p. 66). Even so critical an observer as Chillingworth finds in the minister "high aspiration for the welfare of the race, warm love of souls, pure sentiments and natural piety, strengthened by thought and study, and illuminated by revelation" (p. 130). It is no wonder that the young women of the community were enamored with him: to more than one of them he was "enshrined within the sanctity of her heart, which hung its snowy curtains around his image, imparting to religion the warmth of love, and to love a religious purity" (p. 219). So it was with his parishioner, Hester Prynne, who at one point was most probably one of those adoring young women.

Hester, a person of daring imagination, must have sensed a kindred spirit in Dimmesdale in whom "thought and imagination were so active and sensibility so intense" (p. 124). In addition to her appreciation of his intellect and spiritual qualities, she would have found him, of "striking" appearance with "large, brown, melancholy eyes" (p. 66), a compelling example of vigorous and virtuous young manhood. The contrast with her husband who is repeatedly referred to as both old and deformed, and to whom she had been ensnared in a passionless marriage, is stark indeed. Dimmesdale awakens her hitherto dormant capacity for passion and love. Toward the end of all their trials, the narrator affirms, and, because of its significance, I will refer to the affirmation several times, that he was the man she "once,–nay, why should we not speak it?–still so passionately loved! " (p. 193). Hester fell in love with Dimmesdale for the "invaluable gold" (p. 130) to be found in his heart, mind, and spirit. Everything that she did for him subsequently, including her return to Boston, as we shall see, expresses the profound and enduring nature of her love.

The superlative descriptions of Dimmesdale gainsay Nina Baym's (1986) and a host of other contemporary critics' judgment that, regarding Hester, "We cannot see in Dimmesdale what she sees in him" and that her love for him was a "delusion [...] perhaps purely Hester's creation, built from her desire on the sands of Dimmesdale's weaknesses" (p. 26). Magnus Ullén (2004) draws attention to the several-decades of critical trend to subject Dimmesdale to persistently negative judgments, as if he were "an antagonist of Hester rather than her beloved" (p. 101).[9] Hester herself contradicts Baym and other critics' deprecatory judgments. Seeing him on the scaffold during the night vigil, she apprehends the stark contrast between the man before her and the Arthur Dimmesdale she had known: "*Knowing what this poor, fallen man had once been,* her whole soul was moved by the shuddering terror with which he had appealed to her" (p. 159, emphasis added). If, as these critics assert, Hester's years of love, devotion and sacrifice for Dimmesdale are based on delusion, we might pity but not admire her, nor would she merit the status as the principal female character in our national literature. And the tragedy that haunts the "tale of human frailty and sorrow" (p. 48) thereby becomes depleted of meaning; heroism is founded on clarity of vision, not delusion. Something is amiss here too: if we cannot see what Hester saw, perhaps we need to examine our blindness, not hers. A critical reassessment of Arthur Dimmesdale from a psychoanalytic perspective, the subject of Chapter 2, reveals him to be an admirable, albeit flawed, tragic hero, most worthy to be Hester's beloved. Hester Prynne and Arthur Dimmesdale's fates are deeply intertwined and their tragedies are mutual.

The bond between Hester and Dimmesdale evolved before the romance's opening scene, and as such it is out of the reader's view. Two statements are made by Dimmesdale which intimate the sources of his love for the heroine. In response to her refusal on the scaffold to speak his name as her partner in sin, he whispers, "wondrous strength and generosity of a woman's heart" (p. 68). And, when being revived by her presence in the forest, he professes, "Neither can I any longer live without her companionship; so powerful she is to sustain, –so tender to soothe!" (p. 201). Throughout the text, however, there are many descriptions and judgments from which one can assemble both a larger and more detailed portrait of Hester, one which reveals a person of extraordinary strength of character and conviction, abundant courage, virtue and generosity as well as compelling beauty. Even under the strain of the scaffold she manifests a "natural dignity" and a "force of character" (p. 52). She possessed "a mind of native courage and activity" (p. 199) which she employs toward rigorous self-scrutiny in order to determine if there had been "a defect of truth, courage and loyalty on her part" (p. 166). Her spirit was "strong, calm, stedfastly enduring" (p. 245). As a mother she loved her child "with the intensity of sole affection" (p. 179). I detail her legendary beauty: she possessed a "tall figure of perfect elegance on a large scale, dark and abundant hair...and a face beautiful from regularity of feature, marked brow and deep black eyes" (p. 53). She carried herself with a "certain state and dignity" (p. 53). There was strong sensual aspect to her pulchritude as it emanated from her nature which possessed "a rich, voluptuous, oriental characteristic" (p. 83). Her "taste for the gorgeously beautiful" (p. 83) found expression in the notable artistic creativity of her stitchery, the product of "so much gorgeous and luxuriance of fancy" (p. 53). Despite being compromised by the isolation imposed upon her by the community and harboring resentment toward her oppressors, Hester, in her work as a sister of mercy for the afflicted, showed herself to have an exemplary character and a benevolent spirit worthy of the highest admiration: she was "quick to acknowledge her sisterhood with the race of man, whenever benefits were to be conferred. None so ready as she to give her little substance to every demand of poverty. None so devoted as Hester when pestilence stalked through the town. In all seasons of calamity–whether general or individual, the outcast at once found her place" (p. 160). And, most movingly, in the emergencies of "the sufferer's hard extremity" (p. 160) and impending death, "Hester's nature showed itself warm and rich; a well-spring of human tenderness, unfailing to every real demand and inexhaustible by the largest" (p. 160). Is there any wonder that generations of readers, using their feelings as a guide, find themselves to have fallen in love with Hester Prynne?

The Scaffold of Trauma

The minister knew that Hester was a married woman and that adultery transgresses "one of the most sacred" (p. 200) of received laws. We have Chillingworth's informed assessment that Dimmesdale had "a strong animal nature" (p. 130). However we imagine their sexual relationship, it was comprised of a "single instance" (p. 200) which the narrator characterizes, on Dimmesdale's part at least, as "a sin of passion, not of principle, nor even purpose" (p. 200). The physician was essentially correct that: "He hath done a wild thing ere now, this pious Master Dimmesdale, in the hot passion of his heart!" (p. 137). The reader can imagine that in a secluded encounter, Dimmesdale's "mightier touch [did] awaken all her sensibilities." Hester's "impulsive and passionate nature" (p. 57) combusted with Dimmesdale's "strong animal nature" and the rest is literary history.[10] Pearl and the scarlet letter are its legacies. This is the moment that witnesses the truth of Matthiessen's judgment, "Hester's tragedy came upon her in consequence of excessive yielding of her own heart" (p. 348). However the sexual union evolved, after the Act was the Word. In the forest Hester reminds Dimmesdale of an interchange they had afterward which is the reader's one direct access to the scene: "'What we did had a consecration of its own. We felt it so! We said so to each other! Hast thou forgotten it?...Hush, Hester! said Arthur Dimmesdale...No; I have not forgotten!'" (Vol. 1, p. 195). Hester forces the point that at the time there was mutual assent in action, feeling, thought, and interpretation. In the immediate aftermath, their sexual union was imbued with a quality of private consecration.

The fact that Hester is a married woman and pregnant by a man other than her husband and that Dimmesdale is the pastor of a Puritan congregation are inescapable realities the consequences of which shatter their deep but fragile sentiment of consecration. The consecration cannot endure being flung into the public arena with its glaring scrutiny and communal judgments. Their joy is short-lived and their trials and suffering are only beginning. We witness Hester's trial on the scaffold in just such a public glare.

However happy her childhood or dimly ungratifying her life with Roger Prynne in Amsterdam or undistinguished her time in Boston waiting for his appearance, Hester, with one passionate act, is rendered by society a criminal and outcast. She is a woman in crisis and her life will never be the same. On the "pathway that had been so fatal" (p. 80) which led to the sexual union with Dimmesdale, Hester also encounters a truth which will be expressed by the narrator of *The Marble Faun*: "The firmest substance of human happiness is but a thin crust spread over it...It needs no earthquake to open the chasm. A footstep, a little heavier than ordinary, will serve...to break through the crust, at any moment. By-and-by, we inevitably sink!" (Hawthorne, 1962, Vol. 4, pp. 162–163).

During her pregnancy, she had been in "an impassioned state" (p. 91) and "with wild energy....had fought against her sorrows" (p. 184). Her time in prison, with an infant to care for, must have been an extraordinary challenge to her independent spirit and may account in part for the resistance toward authority that she manifests; Hester would not be the only person whose radicalism was born out of the indignities of incarceration. She was repeatedly subject to interrogation and refused to name her lover. The ornate A she embroidered and was to wear as a sign of shame, becomes, in her hands, a token of defiance as is the "combative energy" (p. 78) that underlies her demeanor on the scaffold. Although, through extraordinary strength she executes "a lurid triumph" (p. 78), we should not underestimate how traumatic was her time on the scaffold as it leaves an indelible scar on her psyche. Public shame is actually not the worst of it.

If Hawthorne indeed has no mercy for Hester, it is surely in the nearly unbearable conflicts to which he subjects his heroine on the scaffold. She is under the relentless exposure to critical public gaze and from the importunate demands of the magistrates that she reveal her partner in sin. A resolute silence has tried their patience: "Woman, transgress not beyond the limits of Heaven's mercy!" (p. 68). Hidden in plain sight, Dimmesdale admits to Hester a failure of courage, surely his tragic flaw, and appeals to her, undoubtedly with ambivalence, to speak for him: "I charge thee to speak out the name of thy fellow-sinner and fellow-sufferer!...Take care how thou deniest to him–who perchance, hath not the courage to grasp it for himself–the bitter, but wholesome cup that is now presented to thy lips!" (p. 67).[11] Chillingworth, whose unexpected appearance in the crowd shocks her, simultaneously demands that she conceal public recognition of him and reveal her paramour as he commands her to "Speak; and give your child a father!" (p. 68). Pressures converge on her in an existential moment of incalculable urgency and perplexity. Hester is a practical as well as courageous woman: she needs to consider what good to anyone would accrue if she pointed the finger of guilt at the minister. Her reasons for keeping silent on the scaffold are surely the same as for keeping the oath of silence regarding her husband's identity. Much later she is explicit to Dimmesdale about her motives: "thy good, –thy life–thy fame, –were put into question!" (p. 193). Chillingworth contends, and with good reason, that the revelation of Dimmesdale's partnership in sin would have resulted in his being "hurled from the pulpit into a dungeon, –thence, peradventure, to the gallows!" (p. 171). The minister was revered for his purity; it is not unlikely that the magistrates would have been harsh in the punishment of such a breach of divine and civil law. Adultery was a capital crime; in Hester's calculation, her silence insured not only that her lover's fame would remain intact, and that he could continue to perform good works as minister for the community, but, above all, that his life would be preserved. Nor is it certain that Hester's punishment would have been altered if she had confessed.[12] Michael Ragussis (1982) emphasizes the long-term baleful influence on Pearl and, as it turns out, also on Dimmesdale, of Hester's refusal to name her child's father; he contends that "the tale's center, then, lies less in the crime of sexual transgression than in the crime of silence" (p.863). However, Ragussis fails to consider, as Hester was forced to, the very real alternative that if Dimmesdale's identity as her partner were exposed, he might have been executed. In charging her with a "crime of silence," the critic has the benefit of retrospect which the heroine could not. With so much at stake, Hester erred on the side of caution.[13] Perhaps Cordelia knew best: "Love and be silent."

"The turmoil, the anguish, the despair" (p. 70) of the scaffold left Hester in a state of extreme nervous excitement. When Chillingworth tends to her agitated condition in the prison cell, she expresses dire longings: "I have thoughts of death...have wished for it,–would have prayed for it, were it fit that such as I should pray for anything." Although she was a commanding presence for three hours on the scaffold, the punishment takes its toll and reduces her to feel unworthy to be alive.[14] With her psyche under siege,

Chillingworth again takes advantage of her vulnerable state and extracts from her an oath of silence as to his identity. Even though it appears to be the only way to protect Dimmesdale, Hester has premonition that in agreeing she has made a compact with the devil. She discovers, much later, that her silence has been instrumental in enabling the physician's prolonged torture of Dimmesdale. It had been a fatal miscalculation as it led to the deterioration and death of the man for whose well-being she had, on the scaffold and afterwards, sacrificed everything.

Thus, for Hester, the scaffold of shame is a scaffold of trauma. In relation to the nightmares experienced by patients suffering from traumatic war neuroses, Freud (1920) was to elaborate the concept of the repetition compulsion: the unconscious is forever fixated on the scene of trauma to which it returns over and over again. Hawthorne anticipated Freud's formulation in a description of this compulsion which has never been surpassed: "But there is a fatality, a feeling so irresistible and inevitable, that it has the force of doom, which almost invariably compels human beings to linger around and haunt, ghost-like, the spot where some great and marked event has given the color to their life-time, and still the more irresistibly, the darker the tinge that saddens it" (pp. 79–80). The scaffold was forever to be such a spot for Hester.

The Strange and Solitary Anguish of Her Life

Through strength of will, Hester courageously endures the trials of the scaffold. Afterwards, however, she must settle down to the indignities of a daily existence imposed upon her as the wearer of the scarlet letter. As the narrator tells the reader, in a marvel of understatement, "the effect of the symbol–or, rather, of the position in respect to society that was indicated by it –on the mind of Hester Prynne herself, was powerful and peculiar" (p. 163). In fact, the effect was psychologically devastating; its most noxious consequence was the near total alienation from human contact that it entailed. There is perhaps no more precise or poignant description of the psychological harm wrought by social exclusion:

> In all her intercourse with society, however, there was nothing that made her feel as if she belonged to it. Every gesture, every word, and even the silence expressed that she was banished, and as much alone as if she inhabited another sphere, or communicated with the common nature by other organs and senses than the rest of human kind. She stood apart from mortal interest, yet close beside them, like a ghost that revisits the familiar fireplace, and can no longer make itself seen or felt, no more smile with the household joy, nor mourn with the kindred sorrow; or should it succeed in manifesting its forbidden sympathy, awakening only terror and horrible repugnance (p. 84).

The companionship and sympathy that Hester needed in order to bear her punishment was denied her from all quarters of the community to which she was the object, for a long time, of covert and overt scorn and malice.

Although she was relied upon for her sewing, she was not engaged to fashion a bride's veil: for such a nuptial adornment, the very touch of her fingers was a pollution. As a penitent seeking comfort in what she hoped would be the welcoming embrace of her congregation at the Sabbath service, she was instead objectified as a lesson in sin.[15] Thus a communal path to God was blocked to her. In his rendering of the Puritan community's treatment of Hester, Hawthorne issues a devastating critique of the "cold, spectral monster" (Vol. 3, p. 55) of abstract principle, in this instance it is religious, which is cruelly insensitive to the exigencies of human circumstance. The result was, for Hester, an isolation and alienation of pathogenic proportions. Colucurcio is accurate in his assessment that Hawthorne urges "the outrage to both human privacy and human conscience perpetrated by the 'unpardonable' Puritan practice of exposure and enforced confession" (p. 481).

Nor is sublimation available to Hester as an avenue of instinctual gratification. Her needlework, at which she excelled, "might have been a mode of expressing, and therefore soothing, the passion of her life. *Like all other joys, she rejected it as sin*" (Hawthorne, 1962, Vol. 1, pp. 83–84, emphasis added). This is an extreme measure taken by the superego against any pleasure afforded by the instinctual life. The narrator gravely prognosticates that trouble is ahead for Hester: "This morbid meddling of conscience with an immaterial matter betokened, it is to be feared, no genuine and steadfast penitence, but something doubtful, something that might be deeply wrong, beneath" (p. 84).[16]

Alone and defenseless as she is, Hester adopts a mask of social compliance which hides defiance and anger intermixed with elements of misanthropy: "she forbore to pray for her enemies; lest, in spite of her forgiving aspirations, the works of the blessing should stubbornly twist themselves into a curse" (p. 85). As a consequence, her inner life and her social persona become dissociated. Hester, then, like Dimmesdale, lives a life of hypocrisy.

Of course, Hester's isolation is not total as she has Pearl's ever present companionship, "[m]other and daughter stood together in the same circle of seclusion from human society" (p. 94). In fact, "Never, since her release from prison, had Hester met the public gaze without her" (p. 93). However, such social isolation produces an unwholesome symbiosis. Hester often relates to Pearl as an extension of herself, a living embodiment of her sin and a mirror in which she sees reflected her own aberrant mental states: "her wild, desperate, defiant mood, the flightiness of her temper, and even some of the very cloud-shapes of gloom and despondency that had brooded in her heart" (p. 91). Hester's plea to the Governor reveals a desperate dependence on Pearl: "God gave me this child! He gave her in requital of all things else which ye had taken from me. She is my happiness....she is my torture. Pearl keeps me here in life...ye shall not take her! I will die first!" (p. 113). However, understandable, Hester's life-defining need for Pearl places a very heavy burden on her child.[17] Moreover, near what is surely a loving core of their relationship, lies the secret of the Pearl's paternity which Hester, forced by circumstance to guard, must deal with evasively if not with frank dishonesty. Pearl suffers from the lack of a father and, all the more so, because of the impenetrable mystery that surrounds his identity. Pearl may be vexed but she is not fooled and her signature recalcitrance enacts revenge against her mother. As Pearl is perhaps a source of torture more often than not, for Hester "Her only real comfort was when the child lay in the placidity of sleep" (p. 93). Hester cannot escape from a punishment which encompasses every aspect of her life.

Hester's Trials and the Fate of Her Sexuality

Undoubtedly in order not to betray their liaison, Hester and Dimmesdale do not allow themselves any interaction. "Lonely as was Hester's situation, and without a friend on earth who dared to show himself" (p. 81) is certainly a reference to Dimmesdale who makes no occasion to present himself to her. "Estranged by fate and circumstance" (p. 190), they follow very different paths which serves to create an ever-widening psychological gap between them. Hester's punishment situates her on the fringe of the community; as a religious leader, the minister remains at its center. In his public role, Dimmesdale cares for his flock; Hester raises Pearl in the seclusion of her cottage. Dimmesdale, who carries the burden of hidden guilt and self-punishment envies what he imagines is the "wholesome cup" of Hester's visible penance; Hester's sin and punishment are inescapably a public matter by which she is debased and always in view of Dimmesdale's social elevation. As a consequence of their enforced separation, they have no access to each other's inner lives and the transformations being wrought over time by the other's unique misery. This gap will be of determinative significance in the aftermath of their crucial interchange in the forest.

In a small settlement it was impossible for Hester not to see the pastor, if only in passing: "But sometime, once in many days, or perchance in many months, she felt an eye –a human eye –upon her ignominious brand, that seemed to give a momentary relief, as if half of her agony were shared. The next instant, back it all rushed again, with still a deeper throb of pain; for, in that brief interval, she had sinned anew. Had Hester sinned alone?" (p. 86). The human eye was Dimmesdale's and the relief she feels by being "together," although only as the object of his gaze, turns to pain because it arouses in her forbidden sexual desire. Although there was no intercourse between them, Dimmesdale was alive in Hester's troubled psyche. There is no relief for Hester in the "strange and solitary anguish of her life" (p. 86): being together with Dimmesdale, however fleetingly, provokes conflict and guilt, not comfort.

Hester's sexual union with Dimmesdale was a statement of her passionate nature; it was not, as some critics contend, an act of rebellion against Puritan authority.[18] Hester's sexual prohibitions arose from internal sources as was the guilt when she transgressed them. As a married Christian woman, raised in "a pious home" (p. 111) and undoubtedly having been taught the tenets of Christian morality, her passion for the minister was a sin and, as for its sexual consummation, "she knew her deed had been evil" (p. 89). [19] Apart from the punishing attitude of the community, Hester somehow has to reconcile within herself her feelings toward both her sin and her partner in it. It is a mighty struggle. Since there were no restrictions placed by the magistrates on her movements, Hester could have ended her punishment by leaving the colony. However, within its confines, including the "scene and pathway that had been so fatal" (p. 80), dwelt the man "she passionately loved." She chooses to endure society's punishment and a tormenting conflict between desire and conscience in order to be near Dimmesdale and thus to keep alive the hope of somehow being together with him again. The fantasy of a union with him, we shall see, retains its potency for the rest of her life.

Under the sway of Puritan orthodoxy, with its over-arching concern for the salvation of the soul, Hester's conflict over sexual desire, of necessity, reverberates in the spiritual realm. The struggle between the forces of good and evil which are central to Milton's allegory is never far from Hawthorne's conception of his characters' psychology; undoubtedly Hawthorne in part chose to set the romance in a time and place when Milton's imagery dominated the literary imagination. Thus, Hester's yielding to sexual desire outside her marriage was a sin for which she knew she needed repent; acknowledging such, she "*told herself [that] [h]ere had been her scene of her guilt and here should be the scene of her earthly punishment; and so perchance, the torture of her daily shame would at length purge her soul, and work out another purity than that which she had lost; more saint-like, because the result of martyrdom*" (p. 80, emphasis added). This is an expression, and an exalted one, of traditional Christian hope for a path to heavenly redemption through purgatorial suffering. Although Hester's faith is subject to marked vicissitudes, this hope will eventually be rekindled and will be a motive to return to the scene of her earlier moral struggle.

However, in staying in Boston, Hester also harbored a secret motive which, as expressed by the narrator in a Miltonian simile, "struggled out of her heart like a serpent from its hole" (p. 80). Even at the cost of the soul's damnation, she longed to renew an unrepentant sexual bond with her lover "in a union that, if unrecognized on earth, would bring them together before the bar of final judgement and make that their marriage-altar for a joint futurity of endless retribution" (p. 80). David Leverenz (1983) astutely interprets this puzzling but crucial passage as expressing "the sacrilegious hope that really impels her heart: to be united with Dimmesdale forever, in hell. A Dante-esque fantasy of condemned love lurks in her depths 'like a serpent'." Indeed, Hester's fantasy transports her and Arthur Dimmesdale into the first circle of Dante's Inferno alongside the guilty pair, Francesca da Rimini and Paolo Malatesta, who are punished together for their adultery in a joint futurity of endless retribution.[20] Thus the narrator is accurate to consider that Hester's conscious resolve to stay in Boston to expiate her sin is "half a self-delusion" for, regarding Dimmesdale, "the passion, once so wild, and even yet neither dead nor asleep [was] but only imprisoned within the same tomb-like heart" (p. 180).

An imprisoned *Eros* is not free to invest the body and spirit with its sensual energies. As the months pass into years, prolonged sexual repression takes a profound toll on Hester's femininity: "there seemed nothing in Hester's face for Love to dwell upon; nothing in Hester's form, though majestic and statue-like, that Passion would ever dream of clasping in its embrace; nothing in Hester's bosom, to make it ever again the pillow of Affection. Some attribute had departed from her, the permanence of which had been essential to keep her a woman" (p. 163). It was indeed "a sad transformation" (p. 163): as a result of her "having lived through...an experience of peculiar severity...the outward semblance of tenderness...was crushed so deeply into her heart that it can never show itself more" (p. 163). The reader can vouch for Hester's having survived a sustained existence "of peculiar severity." The narrator, however, foreshadows yet another transformation, which will take place in the forest scene, by suggesting that Hester "might, at any moment become a woman again, if there were only the magic touch to effect the transfiguration. We shall see whether Hester Prynne were ever afterwards so touched, and so transfigured" (p. 164).

Hester on the Verge

Unimpeded by her own misery, Hester's bounteous spirit, remarkably, finds expression in unobtrusively aiding the sick and dying. In this way, she participates narrowly but deeply in the life of society. Like Dimmesdale, having been brought low by her situation, she can identify with those who suffer most and use this identification for social benefit. However admirable her efforts, and the community felt them to be so, they bring her neither pleasure nor human connection. A potent brew of self-denial and anger prevents Hester from reaping the rewards of her good work. The community, in its "almost benevolence" (p. 162), slowly but inevitably comes to recognize, forgive and take steps to embrace "the woman with the embroidered badge" (p. 162). It might have been a time of rapprochement. However, with the receptive tenderness of her heart "crushed," Hester, proud and scornful, and under the guise of submission and humility, repudiates the community's attempts at affiliation. The narrator recounts that after ministering in the house of an afflicted all night, Hester departs in the morning "without one backward glance to gather up the meed of gratitude'"(p. 162). Although there is abundant justification for her rejecting stance toward the society that inflicted so much harm upon her, nevertheless rejection results in an isolation which doubles in upon itself. Not unlike Dimmesdale, Hester suffers the psychologically destructive consequences of a life virtually devoid of empathic engagement.

The community's punishment had proven to be too harsh and too protracted. Under chronic duress, Hester's "life had turned, in great measure, from passion and feeling, to thought" (p. 164). Her voice may have been silenced, her body subdued and her feminine spirit oppressed, but her mind found liberation in speculation of the most far-reaching kind. The scarlet letter had not done its intended office for it had failed to bring a repentant wearer back securely under the yoke of Puritan law. Instead, it had worked to bring about the opposite result: "The world's law was no law for her mind" (p. 164).

Regarding this freedom of mind, Colacurcio asserts that "in every way it comes to seem the reverse of surprising that radical freedom and awakening female sexuality are inextricably linked" (p. 474) and in a more precise formulation, that "Hester finds no way to affirm the legitimacy of her powerful sexual nature without affirming total anarchistic freedom" (p. 483). However, the text makes clear that the linkage is the inverse of what Colacurcio claims: Hester's radical freedom of mind results from the *repression* of her female sexuality, not its awakening. And when, in the forest scene, her sexuality is revived, radicalism is nowhere to be found in the vision of domestic happiness that she conjures for Pearl: "We will have a home and fireside of our own; and thou shalt sit upon his knee; and he will teach thee many things, and love thee dearly" (p. 212). It would seem that, at the time, Hester's social radicalism follows the fate of *The House of the Seven Gables*' young reformer, Holgrave, who tells Phoebe: "The world owes all its onward impulses to men ill at ease. The happy man inevitably confines himself within ancient limits" (Vol. 2, pp. 306–307).

In the chapter, "Another View of Hester," the reader finds that it is Hester who has also taken another view, and a penetrating one, of the world that surrounds her. Not in Wordsworthian harmony and joy, but in discord, sadness, and with an unquiet eye, Hester nonetheless "sees into the life of things." And from her "estranged point of view" (p. 199) she discerns that in the realms of politics, religion, and the relation between men and women all is in need of thorough reform.

Regarding affairs of state, Hester "imbibed the spirit of the age" in which "men of the sword had overthrown nobles and kings" (p. 164) and "in the sphere of theory, moreover, had overthrown and rearranged the whole system of ancient prejudice" (p. 164). The narrator does not specify what is the theory or historic actions that are being overturned, so we can only conjecture at the content of Hester's meditations about them. Of course, but a few years earlier, Hester had lived in England and undoubtedly was conversant with the diverse currents of political and social dissent that roiled that society. To which of these her mind now had particular doctrinal affinity, the reader is not told.

As a victim of the "cunningly devised.... ever active sentence of the Puritan tribunal" (p. 85), it comes as no surprise that Hester, in the freedom of her imaginings, would have wishes "to undermine the foundations of the Puritan establishment" (p. 165). In this regard, the narrator conjectures that Hester "might have come down to us in history, hand in hand with Ann Hutchinson, as the foundress of a religious sect. She might, in one of her phases, have been a prophetess" (p. 165). [21] These "mights" are qualified by a significant caveat: "but in the education of her child, the mother's enthusiasm of thought had something to wreak itself upon" (p. 165). There is no real drive to action behind Hester's thoughts about reforming the Puritan order since, the narrator adds, with what I would stress is significant irony, that her motivation dissipates in the exercise of educating Pearl. Of course, the issue is moot since Hester did have Pearl; without Pearl there would have been no ostracism, and hence, no resulting radicalism, and for that matter, no *The Scarlet Letter*.[22]

Colacurcio comments that "[l]ike Ann Hutchinson, Hester Prynne, is an extraordinary woman who falls aground of a theocratic and male dominated society" (p. 461). However in terms of their significance to the romance, the differences between these women are more meaningful than their affinities. The historical Hutchinson was a prominent figure whose thoroughly reasoned religious doctrines, although considered heretical by many, were rooted in Christian texts and persuasively argued in public debates. She also enjoyed ample social support which enabled her to command a community of followers. Nor did educating fourteen children diminish the ardor of her active dissent. Hester, who eschewed public attention, was an outcast with no social resources whatsoever. Significantly, the reader is told nothing of what might be Hester's evolving religious beliefs which, as the product of alienation, seem, if anything, to have become more nihilistic than theistic: "she held hardly more reverence than the Indian would feel for the clerical band, the judicial robe, the pillory, the gallows, the fireside or the church" (Vol. 1, p. 199).[23] The world's law from which Hester had been set free was, in fact, Christian law. And having "cast away the fragments of a broken chain" that "united her to the rest of human kind" (pp. 159–160), Hester, I contend, has become unmoored from Christian faith.[24] The estrangement from congregational worship undoubtedly contributed to weakening the bonds to her religion. Whatever freedom of mind she achieves, Hawthorne would have us understand, is purchased at a very high price as it leaves the heroine's soul in peril: "Shame, Despair, Solitude! These had been her teachers, –stern and wild ones, –and they had made her strong, but taught her much amiss" (pp. 199–200). In ultimately following Dimmesdale's path to redemption, which is "illuminated…by higher truth" (p. 203), Hester will re-forge a connection, link by link, to the chain of Christian faith.

Hester's insights which are of particular interest to many contemporary critics concern the social position of women for which the only remedies she could see were extreme: "As a first step, the whole system of society is to be torn down and built anew. Then, the very nature of the opposite sex is essentially to be modified before a women can be allowed to assume what seems a fair and suitable position. Finally…[woman] herself shall have undergone a still mightier change," one which might threaten the "ethereal essence" of "her truest life" (pp. 165–166). [25] Hester thus conceives a vast project for women, and society as a whole, one which Robert Milder (1996) observes is "describing the gender revolution not unlike that of the last thirty years" (p. 10). Hester was a woman centuries ahead of her time. She will retain, until the end of her life, these convictions about the radical changes needed in the position of women in society but, like Holgrave, "when, with the years settling down more weightily upon him, his early faith should be modified by inevitable experience" (Vol. 2, p. 180), so, too, Hester will eventually modify this undertaking by situating it in a thoroughly Christian framework. Albeit a visionary, she was also a realist as she undoubtedly recognized that, given her low and powerless circumstances, reforming women's societal position "was a hopeless task before her" (Vol. 1, p. 165).

As we follow these various flights of Hester's thoughts, it is important to remember that they took form in the isolation of her cottage and found no social expression: they were never invested "in the flesh and blood of action" (p. 164). Notwithstanding the penetrating nature of her enlightened thinking, Hester needs to be passive since hers and Pearl's sustenance and, most urgently, her permission to continue to keep Pearl under her care, granted contingently at the Governor's Hall, are solely dependent on the community and its Elders' good will; she dared not actively oppose them. The disparity between the clarity of Hester's reformist vision and its unrealizability in the field of action is the source of increasing despondence and, ultimately, frank disease: "[her] heart had lost its regular and healthy throb, and wandered without a clew in the dark labyrinth of mind; now turned aside by an insurmountable precipice, now starting back from a deep chasm" (p. 166). As to the question of whether a woman's existence was worth accepting, Hester, in profound resignation, "had long ago decided in the negative" (p. 165); only her child keeps her alive. Out of depression, Hester at times contemplates filicide and suicide: "a fearful doubt strove to possess her soul, whether it were not better to send Pearl at once to heaven, and go herself to such futurity, as Eternal Justice should provide" (p. 166). Freedom of thought has not extricated Hester from an insuperable dilemma of being; rather, it has contributed to it. Not unlike Dimmesdale, she is pressed to the verge of emotional breakdown.

Bercovitch's astringent representation of Hester in the midst of these struggles, I believe, is an example of critical interpretation that streams through the analysis of the mind but evades the sensibilities of the heart. He asserts that in her sense of being a victim and self-conscious manipulation of the townspeople, Hester reveals "an ego nourished by antagonism; self-protected from guilt by a refusal to look inward; using penance as a refuge from penitence; feeding on shame, self pity and hatred; and motivated by the conviction that society is the enemy of the self" (p. 622); moreover, hers is a "misguided rebellion: a wild, self-vaunting independence leading by a ghastly logic of its own to the brink of murder and suicide" (p. 623). By not allowing for the profoundly deleterious psychological consequences wrought by Hester's prolonged suffering, Bercovitch's formulation is an instance of Gross's (1960) judgment that: "much of the criticism of the novel has tended to obscure what is poignantly human in the work" (p. 154).

As fate would have it, Hester is rescued from desperation by an unexpected encounter with Dimmesdale on his night vigil. In seeing, up close, the minister's alarmingly deteriorated condition, her love for and dedication to him are rejuvenated. Dimmesdale espies Chillingworth in the uncanny light of a meteor and, in terror, gasps: "Who is that man, Hester? I shiver at him! Dost thou know the man? I hate him, Hester....Canst thou do nothing for me?" (p. 156). Hester will respond to his urgent appeal and resolves to come to his assistance. This new mission, as it were, provides her with a path forward and out of the seemingly hopeless entrapment of a preternaturally active mind blocked from purposeful outlet: Dimmesdale is "an object that appeared worthy of any exertion and sacrifice for its attainment" (p. 166). Like Miriam in *The Marble Faun*, Hester is a woman revitalized by a mission of love.[26] Hester engages in self-reflection and courageously accepts a large share of responsibility for Dimmesdale's misery at the hands of her husband. With magisterial integrity, she judges herself, too strictly, to have been his "bane and ruin" (p. 173). She wonders if, in agreeing to Chillingworth's oath of silence, there had been "a defect of truth, courage and loyalty, on her part, in allowing the minister to be thrown in a position where so much evil was to be foreboded, and nothing auspicious to be hoped" (p. 166).[27] She also questions if an absorption in her own suffering and a degree of "misanthropy of her own trouble" (p. 193), perhaps derived in part from feeling that Dimmesdale was in a more fortunate situation than she, might have rendered her insensitive to Dimmesdale's ongoing and perilous situation in relation to Chillingworth.[28] Hester's insights help her to bridge their long separation and enable her to understand the forces which have brought him near insanity and death. She now reads his situation with stunning clinical accuracy.

Although always a woman of feeling and thought, Hester becomes a woman of reparative action. Based on what she observes that night, she embarks on a plan to extricate him from Chillingworth's destructive influence. Whatever Hester considers to have been her moral defects regarding the minister, she attempts to redress in a valorous confrontation with Chillingworth and a bold initiative to identify his nemesis to Dimmesdale. These actions, heroic in the risks they entail, break the deadlock, literally and figuratively, of an ever more destructive human predicament. Hester contradicts her own assertion, "there is no path to guide us out of this dismal maze" (p. 173). She, in fact, is the guide who blazes the path out.

Mission of Love

Love and the responsibility that goes with it impel Hester to calculate a crossing of paths with Dimmesdale in the forest. She must reveal to him the long-held secret of her husband's identity, even though her revelation necessitates an admission that she had consented to a deception which had proven to be deeply injurious to him. In the face of all her daunting trials, Hester has never been made more fearful than by the prospect of this confrontation: "And now, rather than have this grievous wrong to confess, she would gladly have lain down on the forest leaves, and died there at Arthur Dimmesdale's feet" (p. 193). [29] Dimmesdale reacts angrily to her disclosure: "Woman, woman, thou are accountable to this! I cannot forgive you!" (p. 194). Bespeaking a degree of emotional dependence that enlightens as well as takes the reader aback, Hester feels that the worth of her life hangs in the balance as she implores her lover's forgiveness: "All the world had frowned on her...and still she bore it all...Heaven, likewise had frowned upon her, and she had not died. But the frown of this pale, weak, sinful, and sorrow-stricken man was what Hester could not bear and live! 'Wilt thou yet forgive me?' she repeats over and over again. 'Wilt thou not frown? Wilt thou forgive?'" (pp. 194–195).[30] Dimmesdale responds to the urgency of the appeal and the irrepressibility of her impassioned embrace: "I do forgive you, Hester....I freely forgive you now" (p. 195). Lest there be any doubt as to whether Dimmesdale was the man Hester "still so passionately loved" (p. 193), her extraordinary vulnerability to his rejection should settle the question. This reunion, when "the soul beheld its features in the mirror of the passing moment" (p. 190), was a matter of life and death for each. I believe that their interchange, involving confession, compassion and forgiveness, is a testament to an abiding love, now re-awakened, which will inform their actions until their deaths.

They face an immediate crisis. The revelation that his physician is Hester's husband and his mortal enemy renders Dimmesdale desperate. Not seeing any alternative, the minister prefers to languish until death rather than return to Chillingworth's domination: "What choice remains to me?...Must I sink down there and die at once?" (p. 196). Dimmesdale's threat of death brings Hester, for the first and only time in the narrative, to tears: "'Alas, what a ruin has befallen thee!' said Hester, with the tears gushing into her eyes. 'Wilt thou die for very weakness? There is no other cause!'" (p. 196). The tears Hester sheds here provide a glimpse at what she is destined to feel when Dimmesdale dies in her arms, an experience which is enclosed in the silence of a narrative gap.

Now taking his turn at utter dependence, Dimmesdale implores Hester for help: "Be thou strong for me!... Advise me what to do!" (p. 196). And so she does. We must remember that Hester's mission was to rescue Dimmesdale from Chillingworth, it was not her intention to urge him to leave the settlement. However, in their interchange she discovers, and to her dismay, that Dimmesdale's torment arises not only from the physician's malevolent designs, but from the hypocrisy involved in being, stained by unconfessed sin as he is, an exalted spiritual leader. Although she had sacrificed, and still would sacrifice so much to preserve his eminent position and his ability to serve the congregation, Hester discovers that his sacred work has not contributed to his "good," but, instead, has been a source of perpetual despair. To her question, "is there no reality in the penance witnessed and sealed by good works? And wherefore should it not bring you peace?" (p. 191), the disquieting answer is emphatically, "No, Hester, no... Not peace...None!–nothing but despair!" (p. 192).

With her agile and resourceful mind, Hester determines that separation from Chillingworth will not suffice: Dimmesdale must be free from the

Puritan community, so she believes, if there is a chance for him to regain health and mental normalcy. Her urging him to flee Boston and take up life elsewhere is forceful and unambiguous, and, when she adds that she will accompany him, irresistible. Hester is indeed strong for him and does advise him what to do; what she advises, however, is a course of action which may be what she determines he needs, but runs contrary to everything he believes. If the truth be told, her persuasion is not by rational argument, but by something akin to mesmeric power: "Is the world then so narrow?' exclaimed Hester Prynne, *fixing her deep eyes on the minister's, and instinctively exercising a magnetic power over a spirit so shattered and subdued, that it could hardly hold itself erect*" (p. 197, emphasis added). Dimmesdale, so reduced, yields: "I can no longer live without her companionship; so powerful is she to sustain, – so tender to soothe!" (p. 201). However, Hester's spell will not sustain the minister's resolve to flee with her. Physically and mentally broken as he is and in a moment of long-sought relief, Dimmesdale is swayed by Hester's imperative, "Let us not look back...The past is gone!" (p. 202). After the murder of the Model in *The Marble Faun*, Miriam will similarly implore Donatello, "Forget it! Cast it all behind you!" (Vol. 4, p. 176). For both couples, however, such an abrogation will not be possible. Every action leaves its indelible mark, Hawthorne would have us know: the past is never gone.

Hawthorne has created an impossible situation for his hero and heroine. Despite their desperate need for each other, within the confines of the "magic circle" of one, solitary hour they cannot construct a bridge of understanding which spans the psychological and moral chasm that has developed between them over seven years. In matters that count for both of them, they are very far apart. Hester misjudges Dimmesdale: because of the years of separation, she is unaware of the intractability of his conflict over guilt, which the reader, having peered into the interior of his troubled heart, knows all too well. Whatever attachment to religious doctrine that Hester may have had is now virtually non-existent. Instead, she "had habituated herself to such a latitude of speculation as was altogether foreign to the clergyman" (Vol. 1, p. 199); Dimmesdale, "on the other hand, had never gone through an experience calculated to lead him beyond the scope of generally received laws; although in a single instance, he had so fearfully transgressed one of the most sacred of them" (p. 200). Their sexual union had been a "single instance" of a "sin of passion"; to leave his congregation now, as Hester proposes, with a woman whose husband is known to him as his physician and cohabitor, would be a sin of both principle and purpose. To "[g]ive up this name of Arthur Dimmesdale," as Hester exhorts him to do, "and make thyself another, and a high one, such as thou canst wear without fear or shame" (p. 198) would condemn him, a "man who by the constitution of his nature [...] loved the truth, and loathed the lie as few men ever did" to another iteration of life as a "remorseful hypocrite" (p. 144). In the emotional rush of this scene, the narrator pauses to ask an incisive question: "But Arthur Dimmesdale! Were such a man once more to fall, what pleas could be urged in extenuation of his crime?" (p. 200). Dimmesdale, in an echo of this question, briefly addresses the theological implications of the proposed action with Hester: "O Thou to whom I dare not lift mine eyes, wilt Thou yet pardon me!" (p. 201). Hester's commanding response is concise: "Thou wilt go!" which she says "calmly, as he met her glance" (p. 201). She casts aside a conflict that lies near the core of Dimmesdale's moral being and reasserts the mesmeric influence of her eyes. Hester may no longer be constrained by Christian law but this is not true of Dimmesdale, who is to be, first and last, "a pure priest, a true religionist, with reverential sentiment largely developed, and an order of mind that impelled itself powerfully along the track of creed, and *wore its passage continually deeper with the lapse of time*" (p. 123, emphasis added). For Hester, the chain of faith appears to have been broken; for the minister, quite to the contrary, "it would always be essential to his peace to feel the pressure of faith about him, supporting, while it confined him within its iron framework" (p. 123). Moreover, Hester does not account for the strength of the minister's attachment to his congregation. He tells her: "Lost as my soul is, I would still do what I may for other human souls! I dare not quit my post, though an unfaithful sentinel" (p. 197). In the aftermath of their encounter, when the minister's spirit is no longer subdued and shattered and when he can contemplate, in the solitude of his study, all that has transpired with Hester and its aftermath, he will situate himself again, and with singularity of purpose, within the iron framework of faith. Hester Prynne and Arthur Dimmesdale are, after all, distinctive human beings, each with outstanding strengths and vulnerabilities. Their fates become irreconcilable.

Needless to say, the strength behind Hester's prompting Dimmesdale to start a new life abroad derives from her own peremptory needs as well as her concern for the minister's welfare. Unconsciously, she has remained in Boston to be near Dimmesdale and, in fantasy, has been willing to endure the flames of Hell in order to forge with him a union, albeit adulterous, "for all futurity." She has suffered extreme isolation and alienation; she has been without assistance in raising Pearl; she has been without a loving partner. So, if, as the narrator suggests, "the whole seven years of outlaw and ignominy has been little other than a preparation for this very hour," Hester is more than ready to join with Pearl and Dimmesdale to "have a home and fireside of our own" (p. 212). This is her chance and she grasps it. She and Dimmesdale have surely, in her words, "ransomed one another, with all this woe!" (p. 256). No reader will deny her that.

The Minister's Transformation

After they part at the verge of the forest, Hester, who will make the arrangements for their passage to Bristol, does not see Dimmesdale until three days later when he appears in the Election Day procession to the Meeting House. She is wounded and "could scarcely forgive him" (p. 240) when he does not give her a glance of recognition as he passes her by. He seems "utterly beyond her reach" (p. 239) and unrecognizable as the man she sat with "hand in hand [as] they mingled sad and passionate talk with the melancholy murmur of the brook. How deeply had they had known each other then! And who was this man? She hardly knew him now!" (p. 239). What Hester does not know, and will not begin to comprehend until he calls her to mount the scaffold with him in a short while, is that the minister is both a transformed and a dying man.

The aberrant exhilaration and effervescent mood that the minister evidences on his return townward derive from having breathed, with Hester, "the wild, free atmosphere of an unredeemed, unchristianized, lawless region" (p. 201). Dimmesdale is released, for a time, from the harsh domination of a punitive superego, with its rigid Puritan cast, which has been surrendered to Hester's liberated conscience.[31] However, all is not well within the minister's psyche as such an abrupt and marked swing out of depression does not bode well. Indeed, Dimmesdale enters a state of mania in which he is flooded with erotic and destructive impulses which he can barely contain. In Dimmesdale's struggle against the instinctual onslaught, he attempts to locate the inciting agent outside himself: "What is it that haunts me and tempts me thus? [...] Am I mad? Or am I given over to the fiend?" (p. 222). However understandable, the decision to succumb again to what, in his Puritan framework, is a life of sin with Hester has poisoned his moral foundation and awakens in him a potential for "Scorn, bitterness, unprovoked malignity, gratuitous desire for ill and ridicule for whatever was good and holy" (p. 222). In a Walpurgisnacht, the dark vault of Dimmesdale's haunted mind has been flung open and he is forced to encounter the twin fiends of *Eros* and *Thanatos* that dwell therein.

As was true of Clifford's manic condition in *The House of the Seven Gables,* the minister's state is "diseased and transitory" (Vol. 2, 258) and extinguishes itself when he re-enters his familiar chamber amidst the stabilizing appurtenances of his hitherto devout Christian life. As he surveys the dwelling, his glance comes upon the Bible and he re-finds, in the moment, his moral compass: "There was the Bible...with Moses and the Prophets *speaking to him*, and God's voice through it all" (p. 223, emphasis added). The Kingdom of God re-establishes its primacy as the minister's moral code; renewed religious devotion will determine everything he does until his death.

Thus begins Dimmesdale's momentous transformation. Having achieved a respite from the lashings of the superego and the urgency of the id, Dimmesdale's ego now exercises considerable powers of self-observation, reflection and integration: "But he seemed to stand apart, and eye this former self with scornful, pitying, but half-envious curiosity. That self was gone! Another man had returned out of the forest; a wiser one; with a knowledge of hidden mysteries which the simplicity of the former never could have reached. A bitter kind of knowledge that!" (p. 223).

The narrator, however, gives no detail as to Dimmesdale's internal processes in this confrontation with himself; like the narrative gap concerning

Hester, Hawthorne has thrown a veil of silence over the minister at a moment of utmost significance, one which "forces us to represent it to ourselves, by ourselves." The nature of the transformation can be read in Dimmesdale's subsequent actions, all contrary to the reader's expectations: the dismissal of Chillingworth as his physician, the composition of an authentic and inspired Election-day sermon, the confession of his sin before the community on the scaffold and acknowledgment of Pearl as his daughter.

In a tense encounter, Dimmesdale cannily frees himself from Chillingworth, even though, as the physician intimates, without his pharmacologic ministrations, death is the likely consequence.[32] Dimmesdale will chose death, if need be, rather than continued subjugation to his tormentor. Having renewed his moral integrity apart from the influences of both Hester and Chillingworth, the minister is readied to be the recipient of heavenly inspiration, "the grand and solemn music of its oracles" (p. 225), as he sets about to write the Election Sermon.

The reader loses track of the minister for three days until Election Day. In this interval Dimmesdale comes to a realization of utmost significance: he is "a dying man" (p. 254). The minster had entered the forest very near death; a brief revival of energy was stimulated by his encounter with Hester. That vital energy has waned; without his physician's medicaments, it appears that the pastor's life can be sustained for only a short time. Everything to be considered, everything to be decided upon and all that follows in the romance must be understood in the light of his awareness of imminent death. For a spiritual, intelligent, and sensitive person such as Dimmesdale, we need only imagine the nature of the meditations in which he attempts to reconcile, as a dying man must, all his past and present experience, and comes to decide how he will conduct the brief remainder of his life. It is a true test of the man he was and the man he became. Even though we do not know these reflections, we do know that they propel him to two final actions: the delivery of the Election Sermon and a public confession of sin on the scaffold. Gerber observes that Dimmesdale "will wrest the initiative from Hester and become the activating force in the story" (p. 87).

Hester is unaware of his disordered state in the forest, the moral reckoning in his study, the terms of his dismissal of Chillingworth, the divine illumination of his sermon, and, through it all, his cognizance of approaching death. This ignorance accounts for her disorientation when she sees him in the procession and makes her ponder: "And who was this man? She hardly knew him now!" (p. 239). Hester will soon learn who is the man he has become. From outside the meeting house, as if a prelude to the scaffold scene, she hears the prosody, not the distinct words, of the minister's Election sermon; its meanings, refracted through her attuned consciousness, concern "passion and pathos" which is communicated to the congregation "in the native tongue of the human heart;" it is "the complaint of a human heart, sorrow-laden, perchance guilty, telling its secret, whether of guilt or sorrow, to the great heart of mankind; beseeching its sympathy or forgiveness, –at every moment, -in each accent, –and never in vain!" (pp. 243–244). This exquisite passage, which evidences Hester's profound, if still unconscious awareness of Dimmesdale's transformation, anticipates not only what is to be the congregation's response to the minister's revelation on the scaffold, but hers, too.

The Scaffold of Sorrow

The minister's sermon, preached in apostolic "words of flame," (p. 248) inspired "awe and wonder" (p. 248) in the congregation, to whom, according to its "united testimony, never had man spoken in so wise, so high, and so holy a spirit" (p. 248). In all this, it was also discerned that their minister was communicating that he was dying: "their minister whom they so loved – and who so loves them all…had the foreboding of untimely death upon him" (p. 249). As his life is rapidly waning, Dimmesdale, with an elemental Puritan belief in an eternal afterlife, needs to purify his soul. He has compounded the sin of adultery with the hypocrisy of silence; both need to be repented through public confession. He struggles against inner resistance to face a dreaded public exposure. In this task, he calls upon Hester for support which she rallies to give "as if impelled by fate, and against her strongest will" (p. 252). With their departure for Bristol only hours away, Hester is undoubtedly mortified by the unexpected turn of events.[33]

In a reference to their encounter in the forest, Dimmesdale confronts Hester with the question: "Is this not better […] than what we dreamed of in the forest?" (p. 254). And in an allusion to her fantasies of filicide and suicide, Hester responds: "I know not! I know not! […] Better? Yea; so we may both die and little Pearl with us!" (p. 254). Hester is angry with Dimmesdale since he has apparently reneged on their agreement. As she is not aware of all that transpired since they parted, he hastens to impart to her the missing crucial information: "For, Hester, I am a dying man" (p. 254). Bringing her and Pearl to the scaffold with him is, in essence, a final act of love and affirmation of their familial bond. It also indicates to Pearl and to the community that she is his daughter. Hester is finally acknowledged as his partner and beloved. No longer obscure outcasts, both are elevated by their intimate association with the Reverend; because of this, their position in the mind of the community undoubtedly will never be the same. Regarding her deception, Hester has told Dimmesdale in the forest that she realized that "a lie is never good, even though death threatens on the other side!" (p. 193). Facing death, the minister has come to the same hard-won wisdom.[34]

Dimmesdale's last words to Hester, of enduring import, are as pastor to parishioner. In a response to her threat of self-destructive action, he reminds her that her fate is in God's hands not her own. As Hester now knows that he is on the verge of death, perhaps viewing eternity, she turns to him as a guide and seer. In a scene of intimacy and intense pathos, as she supports him on her bosom, she appeals to her minister, in a whisper, to tell her if he can foresee a future for them together in the next world. The reader knows the depth of her need to be together with him and what she has been willing to endure to make it possible. The minister issues a final theological judgment against the romantic enchantment in the forest: their act had been a violation, not a consecration, of their souls; as such, he fears, they will not find "an everlasting pure reunion" although, in the end, God is knowing and merciful. Out of a pressing concern for her soul and her future, Dimmesdale instructs Hester to think only of their sin, undoubtedly as a corrective for her having strayed into "the wild, free atmosphere of an unredeemed, unchristianized, lawless region" (p. 201). He offers himself to her as an example: he has come to see that his long torment was instrumental in bringing him to confession, without which his soul would have been lost forever. He then praises God and with his last word to her, "Farewell!," he expires in her arms.

On the scaffold the Reverend enacts for the community and for Hester the spiritual lessons that inhere in a passionate drama of Christian redemption. Those who are onlookers to the scene are transfigured by its instruction: "The multitude, silent till then, broke out in a strange, deep voice of awe and wonder, which could not as yet find utterance, save in this murmur that rolled so heavily after the departed spirit" (p. 257). Some contemporary critics, marked in their skepticism toward Dimmesdale, interpret the Reverend's confession as false, yet another instance of his inveterate hypocrisy. They are wrong: the community that heard the Reverend's words and witnessed his death are, Hawthorne would have us know, the most reliable arbiters of the truth: "the uninstructed multitude...forms its judgment...on the intuitions of its great and warm heart, the conclusions thus attained are often so profound and so unerring, as to possess the characters of truths supernaturally revealed" (p. 127). Hester is at the center of the multitude; her great and warm heart is most transformed of all by what was revealed.

Hester's Return to Boston

Hester's profound and unerring response to the scene of Dimmesdale's death, spanning years in its formulation but only paragraphs in the text is written into her return to Boston. The narrator withdraws attention from Hester as she is contemplating the form of the dead minister in her arms. Contrary to every wish, the man she loved and for whom she has long sacrificed, the man whose bane and ruin she considered herself to have been, the man whose life she tried to save, and the man who is father of her daughter, is gone forever. The dream of escape and a new life together is shattered. His final and portentous message about their sin must resonate discordantly in her ears. The reader can imagine her confusion and pain. The lessons which inhere in Dimmesdale's transcendent scene of death will take time to assimilate. For now, it is enough to appreciate that, on the fateful scaffold, the fabric of her life is once again rent.

Hester must still raise Pearl, a responsibility that has guided her every action. Earlier she had cried out to the Governor, "Pearl keeps me here in life!" (p. 113); for a bereft Hester, this is more true than ever. The narrator tells us that Hester leaves Boston with Pearl shortly after Chillingworth dies, a temporal association that suggests these two events are connected. There is reason to believe that Chillingworth is transformed by the minister's death and has taken seriously his parting admonition, "May God forgive thee!...Thou, too, has deeply sinned!" (p. 256). As did the minister when he confronted death, so it seems, does the physician seek repentance which is expressed in an act of bestowing his fortune upon Pearl; this gives new meaning to his earlier statement: "Thou and thine, Hester Prynne, belong to me" (p. 76). One can wonder, too, if Hester served as an angel of mercy to him when he was dying as penance for the deep injury that adultery had inflicted upon him. Roger Prynne had been a man of decency when Hester married him; her adultery had led to his becoming a fiend; in the face of death, he recovers his humanity, perhaps with her assistance. With his fortune at her disposal, Hester departs Boston to raise Pearl elsewhere. Their silent embarkation suggests that they leave no attachments and they will contact no one in the Puritan community over the ensuing years.

Pearl is transformed by Dimmesdale's actions on the scaffold. With the kiss Pearl bestows upon the minister, "a spell was broken" (p. 256) and her vexing search for her father is ended. The ineffable sadness of losing her father at the moment she finds him brings tears that "were the pledge she would grow up amid human joy and sorrow, not for ever do battle with the world, but be a woman in it" (p. 256). Moreover, "Toward her mother, too, Pearl's errand as a messenger of anguish was all fulfilled" (p. 256). With no secret between them, mother and daughter look forward to a steadfastly honest relationship.

The reader is told none of the details of Hester and Pearl's existence in England, nor, would it seem, for the purposes of the romance, is it necessary. We can assume that, as Hester foresaw, with the "little chaos of Pearl's character" (p. 180) brought into coherence by Dimmesdale's acknowledgment of her, she developed a character marked by "unflinching courage...uncontrollable will...sturdy pride...self respect...[and]...a distain for falsehood" (p. 180); in her is reflected many of her mother's most admirable qualities. It is no surprise, then, that Pearl would have "joyfully entertained that sad and lonely mother by the fireside" in her new home. As tokens of "love and interest" she will send her mother, who adopts a life of poverty, "articles of comfort and luxury...which only wealth could have purchased, and affection could have imagined for her" (p. 262). With an unwavering "look of heedful love" (p. 58), and against all odds, Hester has successfully raised her daughter to be "happy and married" (p. 252). Hester is at a crossroads and is now free to pursue "a more real life for herself" (p. 262). It is the hearth in her cottage in Boston, not Pearl's fireside in a foreign country, that beckons to her as the place to live out that life.[35]

The reader has encountered the phrase "a more real life" in the Custom House referring to the Collector, a brave, old General who, during his reflections on his vigorous life of military engagement, "lived a more real life within his thoughts, than amid the unappropriate environment of the Collector's office" (p. 23). When the narrator is dismissed from his post as Surveyor he, too, will find a more real life as a writer of romance, one which allows him to participate in the "united effort of mankind" (p. 38) and to seek a unique "happiness to live through the whole range of faculties and sensibilities" (p. 40); none of this enlargement was possible when he was "living off Uncle Sam's gold" (p. 39). In pursuit of a more real life, both he and Hester become "a citizen of somewhere else" (p. 44); the narrator follows in the footsteps of his own Hester Prynne who risked everything when she made the daring move to enlist the whole range of her faculties and sensibilities to fulfill a mission in Boston, one which binds her constantly, generously, and lovingly to the united effort of mankind. Need we wonder, as she is about to cross into her cottage once again, "all alone, and all so changed" (p. 261), that, in the liminal moment between the enormity of her past and the uncertainty of her future, she hesitates, if "only for an instant" (p. 262). All her humanity inheres in that instant as does the heroism which propels her through the threshold.

Whatever the years raising Pearl in England brought for her, Hester remains a "sad and lonely mother" (p. 262). It is as if a part of her psyche, fixated in a state of persistent grief, still remains at the traumatic scene of Dimmesdale's death. What the narrator has earlier written philosophically about love is germane to Hester's plight: "*love renders one individual dependent for the food of his affection and spiritual life upon another and leaves the passionate lover... forlorn and desolate by the withdrawal of his object*" (p. 260, emphasis added). As a woman who remains forlorn and desolate and is "burdened with a life-long sorrow" (p. 263), there is the work of mourning still to be done, which, according to the logic of the romance, can uniquely be accomplished around the site of the scaffold, where, it is fitting to reiterate, "her whole orb of life, before and after, was connected with this spot, as with the one point that gave it unity" (p. 244). Hester returns to seek unity and in this quest Arthur Dimmesdale is her guide.[36]

Dimmesdale's last words instruct her regarding "The law we broke! –the sin here so awfully revealed! –let these alone be in thy thoughts!" (p. 256). Hester follows this dictum to the letter of the law, as it were, by reassuming the scarlet letter as an exertion of "her own free will" (p. 263). It is placed in a position, in accordance with Dimmesdale's prescription, where it can always be in her thoughts: "So said Hester Prynne, and glanced her sad eyes at the scarlet letter" (p. 264). The scarlet letter, taken on willingly, is a measure of her attitude toward finally performing, as one of the purposes of her return, what was "yet to be her penitence" (p. 263). Here we find a retort to the narrator's stern query posed earlier in the romance: "Had seven long years, under the torture of the scarlet letter, inflicted so much misery, and wrought out no repentance?" (p. 177). Hester has had the time and distance to reflect upon this question and to meditate on her life as the wearer of the scarlet letter as well as her part in the sad destinies of Dimmesdale and Chillingworth.

As a person to whom "Truth was the one virtue...which...[she] did hold fast through all extremity" (p. 193), I believe, Hester does confront, psychologically, morally and spiritually, the fateful consequences of her "impulsive and passionate nature" and accept herself as both a "victim of her own frailty, and man's hard law" (p. 87). It is therefore consistent with her character that she determines, as she had done previously in relation to the minister, "to redeem her error, as far as it might yet be possible" (p. 167). Like Dimmesdale before her, Hester transmutes what had been the spectacle of penance into the attitude and acts of sincere repentance. Hester internalizes his ideals and makes them her own. In this profound way, a consequence of mourning, they are enduringly together once more.[37]

Despite all her past good deeds as a sister of mercy, Hester had remained alienated from the community, because in this charitable role, "the world's heavy hand ordained her, when neither the world nor she looked forward to this result. The letter was the symbol of her calling" (p. 161). The role was imposed by the scarlet letter, it was not motivated from within. Indeed, Hester came and went from houses of need with no record in the text of any words exchanged with the people to whom she ministered nor any relationships that developed in the exercise of her calling. When she is no longer compromised by internal conflict over guilty passion nor by the harmful psychological effects of enforced isolation, Hester's innately generous personality has more ample freedom to flourish in ways not possible earlier. With the voluntary assumption of the scarlet letter, Hester's relationship to society changes radically. The letter does not define her role, it is she who defines the letter's new office. And, in acceptance of her sin and in her ongoing penitence, she is uniquely qualified as a guide, counsel and comfort to women who had been subject to any of the various trials of "wounded, wasted, wronged, misplaced, or erring and sinful passion" (p. 263). With the scarlet letter on her breast, these women need feel no shame in Hester's presence. The engagement flows directly from herself to other sufferers and is not filtered through an inauthentic mask of humility which hides scorn and rejection. Hester is re-working the trauma of her past, with all the "bitter kind of knowledge" (p. 223) she derived from it, into reciprocal involvement and social good. She had anguished severely because there had been no one for her to turn to; Hester situates herself as a living resource for women who are enduring similar trials in ways that will mediate and lessen their isolation and suffering. Those who turn to her need not be "alone in the world." As "the champion of some practicable cause" (Vol. 2, p. 181), Hester stands as "a well-spring of human tenderness, unfailing to every real demand and inexhaustible by the largest" (p. 161). It is difficult to overestimate the uniqueness and significance of this accomplishment. Two decades abroad, in vastly different circumstances, and with the "solid wisdom" (p. 238) that comes with time and "sad-colored experience" (p. 238), find Hester's "early faith should be modified" (Vol. 2, p. 80). It is not her purpose to rebel against Puritan society; Hester comes to heal the soul, not the body politic.[38]

In all of this, Hester "had no selfish ends, nor lived in any measure for her own profit and enjoyment" (p. 263). There becomes a saintly quality to her existence which defines the "toilsome, thoughtful and self-devoted years" (p. 263) that made up the remainder of her life. She is very changed from the passionate woman of two decades earlier. Hester no longer believes that she is fated to be a prophetess for women; it will suffice to be their interlocutor and practical guide. Hers is a life of acceptance of the limitations that her sin imposed on her and is part of her mourning for what was lost and can never be realized. Moreover, every aspect of her life in Boston indicates that Hester has taken to heart the religious guidance Dimmesdale imparted to her on the scaffold. James Ellis takes note that "Hawthorne speaks of Hester in terms that would suggest she is now firmly within the Christian scheme" and, further, considers that "in her new role she functions as a kind of female John the Baptist" (p. 58).[39] Edward Wagenknecht (1989) finds that "through Hawthorne's art, [Hester] fulfills the mission of divine and mysterious truth" (p. 94). In her identification with the minister, her life, too, comes to embody "a reverential sentiment largely developed" (p. 123). By returning to the "scene of her guilt" (p. 80), Hester can make real what she had told herself earlier was the reason to stay in Boston, that is, to "purge her soul, and work out another purity than that which she had lost; more saint-like, because of the result of martyrdom" (p. 80). Day after day, and for many years until her death, she toils devotedly to this end; hers is a life lived, it is not a gesture or symbol. At the same time, Hawthorne acknowledges his debt to Spenser, Milton, and Bunyan by enshrining his heroine in an allegory of the progression of the soul.

Hester's devotion finds particular expression in spiritual guidance to women in despair. "So said Hester Prynne," (p. 264) the narrator inscribes, as her precise words are finally brought back to the reader in the romance's last paragraph. These words show Hester to be sharing with her sisters an understanding of the underlying cause of their misery and its corrective: "to establish the whole relation of man and woman on a sure ground of mutual happiness" (p. 263). Her analysis retains its radical quality as it necessitates a total change in social attitudes and structures. Hester comforts her interlocutors with the assurance that, in time, God's truth will be revealed and then, it is her belief, the change that is needed will take place. Hester has come to accept what will be articulated by Hawthorne a year later in *The House of the Seven Gables:* "God is the sole worker of realities" (Vol. 2, p. 180). This conviction does not render Hester passive as she unflaggingly does her part to improve the lot of women. In this, she surpasses "the truest test of a life successful to such an end" (p. 263).[40]

Thus Hester does not "abandon her heroic independence," as Bercovitch concludes; the more real life she pursues in the Bay Colony expresses its fullness. Nor is there a hint of more real life in Greven's (2014) interpretation that Hester has returned to "haunt the haunting precincts of her own ruined and ruining desire" where she "fetishistically" pins the A on her bosom as a sign of the "depth of [her] obsessive, even frightening sexual need" (p. 202). The decades-long remainder of her life in Boston constitutes, for Greven, "her lonely erotic vigil for Arthur" (p. 222). I cannot concur with him that such an existence could be lauded as a radical "reaffirmation of her desire" (p. 206) but, instead, it would be a life bereft of meaning in a frozen posture of masochistic surrender.

As Dimmesdale had demonstrated when "the spirit of prophesy was upon him" (p. 249), Hester also evidences, in her guidance, that she had been inspired by a divine enlightenment regarding "the coming revelation" (p. 263) which allows her to intimate the Second Coming of Christ and, most daringly, to impart to her flock that a woman will be its angel and apostle.[41] A vision of the apocalypse had been prefigured to both Hester and Dimmesdale on the night vigil when, in the unearthly light of a meteor, "They stood in the noon of that strange and solemn splendor, as if it were the light that is to reveal all secrets, and the day-break that shall unite all who belong to one another" (p. 154). And while it is true that Hester, in her humility, believes that she is not destined to be the "angel and apostle" of that revelation, might I have the audacity to take exception to her conviction? The transformations of consciousness that the tale of a woman of wondrous strength and generosity who was alone in this world have both uniquely and universally inspired bear witness that Hester Prynne has become, for our generation in particular, more of a prophetess than either she, or perhaps Hawthorne could have imagined. *The Scarlet Letter* has done its office.

In these aspects of her new life in Boston, Hester shows herself to be a transformed woman. The scene of Dimmesdale's death has informed the spiritual life of all who participated in it. Dimmesdale's name does not appear in the epilogue of the romance but it is his loss that defines Hester "as a woman burdened with a life-long sorrow" (p. 263). She returns to Boston to bear her burden and live out her destiny with the dignity and courage worthy of a tragic heroine: it is her crowning development. And it is this Hester Prynne whose history is recorded from oral testimony by Surveyor Pue, where is she is described as a woman "who gained from many people the reverence due to an angel" (p. 32).[42] And the frayed and defaced scarlet A that is discovered by the narrator with the manuscript is last worn by her as the saintly, not sinning, woman. And it is this Hester Prynne that the community, prompted by "the intuitions of its great and warm heart" (p. 127), deems worthy to be buried in her rightful place next to the revered Arthur Dimmesdale. That they are united, but only in death, constitutes the essence of their tragic destiny.

The unconscious, too, has its say in Hester's return. It is the nature of the traumatized psyche to return over and over to the site of trauma. This characteristic defines the still unraveled mystery of Freud's repetition compulsion. So Hester, along with the motives which derive from the knowledge and wisdom of her consciousness, is also drawn by the unconscious to return to the scaffold; in this we bear witness to the truth which, in the end, is itself worthy of repetition: "there is a fatality, a feeling so irresistible and inevitable that it has the force of doom, which almost invariably compels human beings to linger around and haunt, ghost-like, the spot where some great and marked event has given the color to their lifetime; and still the more irresistibly, the darker the tinge that saddens it" (pp. 79–80). In returning to Boston, Hester has responded to this "irresistible and inevitable" call.

Notes

1. Quoted in Lawrence E. Sganlon (1962). In the Introduction to *The Nigger of the Narcissus*, Joseph Conrad memorably express a similar literary ethos: "A work that aspires, however humbly, to the condition of art should carry its justification in every line. And art itself may be defined as a single-minded attempt to render the highest kind of justice to the visible universe, by bringing to light the truth, manifold and one, underlying its every aspect" (p. viii). *The Scarlet Letter*, in my opinion, is an exemplar of Conrad's rigorous standards.
2. Sylvie Mathé's article is an outstanding analysis of the romance's narrative style.
3. Pearl is seven years old at the time of Dimmesdale's death; about a year later, shortly after Chillingworth's death, she departs Boston with her mother at approximately age eight. Hester returns when Pearl, having matured from childhood to womanhood, is married. Although the reader is not told Pearl's age, the interim is referred to as "many years" (Vol 1., p. 261) during which "[the] story of the scarlet letter grew into a legend" (p. 261). One can estimate that the transformation of recent community memory to legend took a substantial part of a generation or twenty years to effect. Therefore, for the remainder of the essay I will employ the phrase "two decades" or "twenty years" as an approximation of the interval between Hester's departure from Boston and her return.
4. Mathé agrees with Bercovitch that, "The effect of such a gap in the narrative is a blurring of reality in which speculation comes to replace information" (p. 611).
5. Reynolds interprets this description of her native dwelling as suggesting Hester's family's links to English aristocracy; this is certainly consistent with her aristocratic bearing (pp. 90–91).
6. The narrator agrees with Hester's judgment of the deleterious impact on her husband: "he [Chillingsworth] was next to treat with her as the man whom she had most deeply and irreparably injured" (p. 73).
7. I agree with this contention by Ellis.
8. Daniel J. Boorstin (1965) states that "[the] applicants for church membership had to satisfy the Elders and then the whole congregation of 'the worke of grace upon their soules, or how God hath beene dealing with them about their conversion...that they are true beleevers, that they have been wounded in their hearts for their originall sinne, and actuall transgressions, and can pitch upon some promise of free grace in the Scripture, for the ground of their faith, and that they finde in their hearts, drawne to beleeve in Christ Jesus, for their justification and salvation...and that they know competenty the summe of Christian faith'" (p. 25).
9. Commentaries too numerous to count confirm Ullén's assertion. For example, Patricia Dunlavy Valenti considers Dimmesdale a man whose "impotencies— sexual, emotional, moral, and verbal—infiltrate every area of his

life" (p. 24) and conjectures that his deterioration is not due to guilt over adultery, but to the practice of "habitual masturbation." David Leverenz (1983) avers that Hester "did not realize how grossly inadequate a man Dimmesdale turns out to be, as a lover, parent and friend" (p. 560). In the same vein, Michael Dunne (1978) comments, "One might easily wonder what it is that Hester sees in the spineless clergyman" (p. 34)

10. D.H. Lawrence (1964), in his famously jaunty commentary on *The Scarlet Letter*, opines that "When Hester Prynne seduced Arthur Dimmesdale, it was the beginning of the end...she tickled him in the right place, and he fell" (p. 89). Moreover, "The greatest triumph a woman can have, especially an American Woman, is the triumph of seducing a man: especially if he is pure" (p. 88). Whatever one thinks of Lawrence's speculations, I submit that Hester, a recent immigrant, was an English, not an American, Woman.
11. This phrase is borrowed from the title of Michael T. Gilmore's 2001 essay, "Hidden in Plain Sight: The Scarlet Letter and American Legibility."
12. In the Bay Colony in 1643, a year encompassed by the chronology of *The Scarlet Letter*, James Britton and Mary Latham were executed for adultery (Newberry, 1987, p. 260). As for Hester's sentence, Reverend Wilson holds out the possibility of removing the scarlet letter if she names her partner in sin: "Speak out the name! That, and thy repentance, may avail to take the scarlet letter off thy breast" (Vol. 1, p. 68). It is also conceivable that her punishment, considered by some of the women in the crowd to be uncommonly lenient given her crime, might have become more severe if it turned out to be their spotless pastor whom she had seduced to entertain Satan with her.
13. Leland S. Person, Jr. (1989) contends that Hester's silence in response to Dimmesdale's appeal to name him is tantamount to her joining with Chillingworth in a plot of revenge against him. Even a psychoanalyst would be loathe to make such an uncharitable interpretation.
14. Death wishes will recur later as the product of seven years of isolation.
15. "If she entered a church, trusting to share the Sabbath smile of the Universal Father, it was often her mishap to find herself the text of the discourse" (Vol. 1, p. 85). Although for different reasons, in *The House of the Seven Gables*, Hepzibah and Clifford are isolated from their congregation and suffer similar adverse consequences as Hester.
16. In *The Marble Faun*, Miriam's guilty conscience, like Hester's, bars her experience of pleasure: regarding Donatello's affection, she "became sensible of a delight and grief at once, in feeling the zephyr of a new affection with its untainted freshness, blow over her weary, stifled heart, which had no right to be revived by it. The very exquisiteness of the enjoyment made her know that it ought to be a forbidden one" (Vol. 4, p. 82).
17. Charles Swann (2007) incisively comments that by making Pearl "the living hieroglyphic" (p. 68) of her sin, Hester replicates the way that Puritan authorities have depersonalized her as the wearer of the scarlet letter. He adds, "It is only with Dimmesdale's public confession that Pearl can become fully human and escapes from the narrowness and distortion inherent in symbolic identity" (p. 68).
18. I do not agree with Seymour L. Gross's (1960) assertion that "Hester's sense of guilt can only be related to what she had done to her lover...she has committed no evil in terms of her own morality" (p. 159). My view accords

with Baym's (1990): "The sexual encounter which forms that donnée of *The Scarlet Letter* was an act neither of deliberate moral disobedience, nor of conscious social rebellion" (p. 209).

19. It is not clear why John C. Gerber (1988) concludes that "God has never been a very real presence in [Hester's] life" (p. 73). Although her faith eventually weakens before it is renewed, for the first years of her punishment Hester was in significant conflict about what she knew was a sin against God's law.
20. Hawthorne's tale also resonates with Boccaccio's telling of the legend in *The Decameron:* Francesca is tricked into marrying Giancotto, the disfigured brother of her betrothed, Paolo. The guilty lovers are killed by Giancotto and buried in a single tomb.
21. It was not just the narrator who thinks so; as we find out later, Hester did, at some earlier moment in time, "imagine that she herself might be the destined prophetess" (Vol. 1, p. 263).
22. Thus, it is not as Colacurio (1972) contends, "the tale and the teller" that "force [Hester] to abandon those [antinomian} conclusions" but the presence of little Pearl. Pearl exerts a dampening influence again in the forest when she insists that her mother resume wearing the scarlet letter which she had impulsively discarded.
23. Colacurcio notes the lack of information regarding Hester's creeds: "to be sure, *The Scarlet Letter* details items of Hester's beliefs even less than the early sketch specifies those of Mrs. Hutchinson" (p. 479).
24. Earlier in the romance, Hester's faith shows what might be signs of wavering: regarding Pearl, she exclaims, "O Father in Heaven,–if Thou art still my Father, –what is this being which I have brought in to the world!" (p. 96).
25. Holgrave, in *The House of the Seven Gables*, is another visionary at the margin of society who, not unlike Hester, advocates that "the moss-grown and rotten Past is to be torn down, and lifeless institutions to be thrust out of the way, and their dead corpses buried, and everything to begin anew" (Vol. 2, p. 179). Also like Holgrave, Hester's vision involves changes in social institutions that are not associated, in its early iteration, with religious awakening. For Hester, that will come later.
26. In several respects, the dilemma that Miriam articulates in *The Marble Faun* resonates with Hester's: "my too redundant energy is slowly–or perhaps rapidly–wearing me out, because I can apply it to no use" (Vol. 4, p. 280). Miriam also rediscovers a purpose in devoting herself to assisting the man she loves and feels she has harmed: "If Donatello is entitled to aught on earth, it is to my complete self-sacrifice for his sake. It does not weaken his claim, methinks, that my only prospect for happiness (a fearful word, however) lies in the good that may accrue to him from our intercourse" (Vol. 4, p. 283). Hepzibah, in *The House of the Seven Gables*, is another of Hawthorne's heroines who finds meaning and purpose in dedication to a man: "I devote myself to Clifford. He has every comfort which his situation admits of" (Vol. 2, p. 226).
27. To be fair, when Hester took the oath, Chillingworth was ignorant of her lover's identity. At that time she could have had no idea that her husband would pursue and torment him. She did come to know that they lived together; here is where she finds reason to admonish herself for having failed to imagine the evil that could be visited upon Dimmesdale in this position.

28. These reflections, which Gerber characterizes as "cuttingly honest" (p. 84), undercut Bercovitch's contention that Hester was "self-protected from guilt by a refusal to look inward" (p. 622).
29. Dimmesdale's state of despair immediately before the encounter is expressed in similar terms as Hester's: "There was a listlessness in his gait; as if he saw no reason for taking one step further, nor felt any desire to do so, but would have been glad, could he be glad of any thing, to fling himself down at the root of the nearest tree, and lie there passive for evermore" (Vol. 1, p. 188).
30. Brook Thomas (2004) points out that Miriam, in the scene in the Marble Saloon in *The Marble Faun*, displays a similar vulnerability to Donatello's possible rejection (p. 178): "this proud and self-dependent woman has wilfully flung herself, hanging her life upon the chance of an angry or favourable regard from a person who, a little while before, had seemed the plaything of the moment" (Vol. 4, p. 283).
31. The mechanism of identifying or yielding the superego with that of another person or persons is described by Freud in "Group Psychology and the Analysis of the Ego."
32. Chillingworth tried to instill fear in Dimmesdale: "Were it not better... that you use my poor skill tonight?...The people look for great things from you; apprehending that another year may come about, and find their pastor gone." Dimmesdale replies: "Yea, to a better world" (Vol. 1, p. 324).
33. There are critics who do not react with "awe and wonder" to the Reverend's final actions. Colacurcio considers the words of flame of the sermon to have been preached "in bad faith" (p. 493). In an overwrought rhetoric, Michael Pringle (2007) issues a denunciation of Dimmesdale: "in a stunning final act of betrayal, Arthur attempts to take from Hester the symbol she has worked seven years to make her own...in belatedly claiming his shame, Arthur reinvokes the stigma on Hester with nearly its original fixity and then leaves her to bear it alone, worn down, humiliated, betrayed and deserted; Hester finally breaks. Unable to live any longer with the Puritans, or apart from community, Hester ends her resistance and flees to Europe with Pearl" (p.48). On the other hand, Dennis Forster (1983) contends that Dimmesdale, manipulating rhetoric to the end, does not confess to anything.
34. David Greven (2016) considers Dimmesdale to be "the cowardly, wholly self-involved man who "preserves his spiritual life at the cost of her [Hester's] happiness and her dignity" (p. 209) and who rejects her with "terrible finality" (p. 221) by "choos[ing] death over love and sex" (p.200) with her. Condemnations of this kind result from a failure to appreciate the truths that Hester has to confront: Dimmesdale is a transformed and dying man. "That self was gone!" Without this appreciation, Hester's return to Boston is wholly unintelligible.
35. It is not clear, as Bercovitch imagines, that there was a "a dramatic moment when Hester decides to come home to America" (p. 631). The decision may have been a long time in contemplation but could not be acted upon until Pearl was independent. Moreover, I do not think it apt to refer to Hester as coming "home to America." Hester was raised in England, spent time in Amsterdam as a married woman, and lived seven years as a pariah in inhospitable Boston. She then returns "home" to England for two decades. There is no reason to believe that she made a "patriotic" attachment to the colony and thought of herself as coming "home to America" in that sense. The ties to England were strong; in the 1648 Cambridge Platform the

ministers declared: "wee desire not to vary from the doctrine of faith, & truth held forth by the churches of our native country...wee, who are by nature, English men" (Boorstin, 1965, p.16.)

36. Herein lies the answer to the question that perplexes Bercovitch (1991): "the entire novel tends toward this moment of reconciliation, but the basis for reconciliation, the source of Hester's revision remains entirely unexplained" (p. 2). Bercovitch can conclude that Hester "chooses for no clear reason" to return to Boston because his analysis excludes an examination of her psychology, a hazardous omission regarding a psychological novel. Instead, he imposes an abstract concept of her "being an exemplar of continuity through integration" as her putative motivation. I contend that such a consideration was foreign to Hester and would never have passed through her mind during "her unrecorded period of self-scrutiny in the old world." Nor do I believe it was Hawthorne's purpose to deploy his heroine as a means to "urge gradualism and consensus" as a democratic imperative; in the Preface to *The House of the Seven Gables*, Hawthorne makes clear that regarding the ending of a romance: "The Author has considered it hardly worth his while, therefore, relentlessly to impale the story with its moral, as with an iron rod" (Vol. 2, p. 2).
37. Hester follows in the footsteps of Arthur Dimmesdale much more than she ever did those of Ann Hutchinson. In "Mourning and Melancholia," Freud elaborates the concept of identification with the lost object as part of the process of mourning.
38. Greven (2014) contends that there are "important tensions that exist in the scenes between the returned Hester and the women who seek her counsel" (p. 205). He states that Hester, still struggling with sexual desire, "manipulates her thoughts and fights against too volatile and threatening and transgressive ones" (p. 205) so as to conceal from these women the "war between what she must feel and what she does feel" (p. 205). There is no support in the text for these assertions; a psychoanalyst must step in to correct the record here. Counselling that is consequential, as undoubtedly Hester's was, demands as close an alignment as possible between the counsellor's feelings and words. Anything less is ineffective therapeutically as it is, in essence, an exercise in hypocrisy. In the intervening decades, a mature Hester has grown beyond the "half a self-delusion" (Vol. 1, p. 80) that characterized a repression of awareness of sexual desire when she was living in proximity to Dimmesdale. For that was in another era. And besides, the minister is dead.
39. Ellis (1980) underscores that Hester's sacred vision of the future, concerning the new relation of man and woman, is "vertical and microcosmic" and is complementary to the one revealed by Dimmesdale in the Election Sermon, which is "horizontal and macrocosmic." The reconciliation of the two, Ellis believes, can be found within the fulfillment of the sacrament of matrimony on earth while anticipating redemption together in heaven. Hawthorne touchingly expresses this vision in a letter to his bride, Sophia Peabody: "Shall I not hold you in my arms when we are angels together?"
40. My interpretation also disagrees with that of Jamie Barlowe (2000) who contends that by replacing the scarlet letter, Hester may change its signification but "in order to do so, she must now admit her own sin and shame, giving up her dreams and her voice in service of the community" (p. 7).
41. Swann (2007) points out that the coupling of revelation with the words "angel and apostle...makes the millenarian nature of Hester's prophecy quite clear" (p. 78) and further, "it looks like Hester expects a lot: the

Second Coming" (p. 79). In the face of what is Hester's prediction of the total transformation of the relationship between man and woman, Swann cannot accept Bercovich's concept of reconciliation and compromise: "to argue that Hawthorne speaks from and celebrates an ideology of liberal consensus seems entirely wrong" (p. 80). Michael Davitt Bell sees Hester in the tradition of her biblical namesake, Esther, a "homiletic example of sorrow, duty and love" (Bercovitch, p. 176).

42. When Hester was "very old" (Vol. 1, p. 32) she retained a "stately and solemn aspect" (p. 32); undoubtedly she was afforded a reverence which, as in the times of the early settlers, was "bestowed...on the white hair and venerable brow of age; on long-tried integrity; on solid wisdom and sad-colored experience; on endowment of that grave and weighty order, which gives the idea of permanence, and comes under the general definition of respectability" (pp. 237–238).

References

Abbott, A. (1988). The Magic Power of Hawthorne's Style. In D. Kesterson (Ed.), *Critical Essays on Hawthorne's The Scarlet Letter.* G.K. Hall.

Barlowe, J. (2000). *The Scarlet Mob of Scribblers: Rereading Hester Prynne.* Southern Illinois University Press.

Baym, N. (1986). *The Scarlet Letter: A Reading.* Boston: Twayne Publishers.

Baym, N. (1970). Passion and Authority in *The Scarlet Letter. The New England Quarterly*, 43.

Bell, M. (1975). Hawthorne and the American Romance. In S. Bercovitch, *The Puritan Origins of the Self.*

Bercovitch, S. (1988). The A-Politics of Ambiguity in *The Scarlet Letter. New Literary History, 19*(3), 631.

Bercovitch, S. (1991). *The Office of the Scarlet Letter.* Johns Hopkins University Press.

Bloom, H. (2004). *Bloom's Major Literary Characters: Hester Prynne.* (H. Bloom, Ed.) Chelsea House.

Boorstin, D. (1965). *The Americans: The Colonial Experience.* Vintage Books.

Brown, G. (1991). Hawthorne, Inheritance, and Women's Property. *Studies in the Novel, 23*(1).

Buell, L. (2014). *The Dream of the Great American Novel.* Cambridge: Harvard University Press.

Carpenter, F. (1988). Scarlet A Minus. In D. B. Kesterson (Ed.), *Critical Essays on Hawthorne's The Scarlet Letter.* Boston: G. K. Hall.

Chodorow, N. J. (1999). *The Power of Feelings.* New Haven: Princeton.

Colacurcio, M. (1972). Footsteps of Ann Hutchinson: The Context of *The Scarlet Letter. ELH*, 39(3).

Conrad, J. (1921). *The Nigger of the Narcissus: A Tale of the Forecastle.* New York and Toronto: Doubleday, Page & Co.

Cottom, D. (1982). Hawthorne Versus Hester: The Ghostly Dialectic of Romance in *The Scarlet Letter. Texas Studies in Literature and Language, 24*(1).

Dunne, M. (1978). Hawthorne, the Reader, and Hester Prynne. *Interpretations, 10*(1).

Ellis, J. (1980). Human Sexuality, the Sacrament of Matrimony, and the Paradox of the Fortunate Fall. *Christianity and Literature*, *29*(4).

Forster, D. (1983). The Embroidered Sin: Confessional Sin in *The Scarlet Letter*. *Criticism*, *25*(2), 141–163.

Freud, S. (1920). Beyond the Pleasure Principle. In J. Strachey, A. Freud, A. Strachey, & A. Tyson, (Trans.), *Standard Edition*. (Vol. 7, pp. 65–134) London: Hogarth.

Freud, S. (1921). Group Psychology and the Analysis of the Ego. In J. Strachey, A. Freud, A. Strachey, & A. Tyson, (Trans.), *Standard Edition* (Vol. I8, pp. 65–134). London: Hogarth.

Freud, S. (1959). Mourning and Melancholia. In J. Strachey (Ed.), *The Standard Edition of the Complete Psychological Works of Sigmund Freud* ((J. Strachey, Trans., pp. 243–258). Hogarth Press and the Institute of Psycho-Analysis.

Gerber, J. (1988). Form and Content in *The Scarlet Letter*. In D. Kesterson (Ed.), *Critical Essays on Hawthorne's The Scarlet Letter*. G.K. Hall.

Gilmore, M. (2001). Hidden in Plain Sight: *The Scarlet Letter* and American Legibility. *Studies in American Fiction*, *29*(1).

Greven, D. (2016). *Gender Protest and Same-Sex Desire in Antebellum American Literature*. London and New York: Routledge.

Gross, S. (1960). Solitude, and Love, and Anguish: The Tragic Design of *The Scarlet Letter*. *CLA Journal*, *3*(3).

Hawthorne, N. (1962).*The Blithedale Romance*. In W. Charvat (Ed.), *The Centenary Edition of the Works of Nathaniel Hawthorne* (Vol. 3). Columbus: Ohio State University Press.

Hawthorne, N. (1962).*The House of the Seven Gables*. In W. Charvat (Ed.), *The Centenary Edition of the Works of Nathaniel Hawthorne* (Vol. 2). Columbus: Ohio University State Press.

Hawthorne, N. (1962). *The Marble Faun*. In W. Charvat (Ed.), *The Centenary Edition of the Works of Nathaniel Hawthorne* (Vol. 4). Columbus: Ohio State University Press.

Hawthorne, N. (1962).*The Scarlet Letter*. In W. Charvat (Ed.), *The Centenary Edition of the Works of Nathaniel Hawthorne* (Vol. 1). Columbus: Ohio State University Press.

Lawrence, D. (1964). *Studies in Classic American Literature*. Viking Press.

Leverenz, D. (1983). Mrs. Hawthorne's Headache: Reading *The Scarlet Letter*. *Nineteenth-Century Fiction*, *37*(4).

Lewis, R. (1955). *The American Adam*. University of Chicago.

Mathé, S. (1992). The Reader May Not Choose: Oxymoron as Central Figure on Hawthorne's Strategy of Immunity from Choice in *The Scarlet Letter*. *Style*, *26*(4).

Matthiessen, F. O. (1941). *American Renaissance: Art and Expression in the Age of Emerson and Whitman*. New York: Oxford University Press.

Milder, R. (1996). *The Scarlet Letter* and Its Discontents. *Nathaniel Hawthorne Review*, *22*(1).

Newberry, F. (1987). A Red-Hot Lusting Divine: Sources for *The Scarlet Letter*. *The New England Quarterly*, *60*(*2*).

Person, L. Jr. (1989). Hester's Revenge: The Power of Silence in *The Scarlet* Letter. *Nineteenth-Century Fiction*. *43*(4). 465–483.

Pringle, M. (2007). The Scarlet Lever: Hester's Civil Disobedience. *ESQ: A Journal of the American Renaissance*, *53*(1).

Ragussis, M. (1982). Family Discourse and Fiction in *The Scarlet Letter*. *ELH*, *49*(4).

Reynolds, L. (1988). *European Revolutions and the American Literary Renaissance*. Yale University Press.

Sandeen, E. (1962). *The Scarlet Letter* as a Love Story. *PMLA*, *26*(4).

Sganlon, L. (1962). The Heart of *The Scarlet Letter*. *Texas Studies in Literature and Language*, *4*(2).

Stanton, R. (1970). *The Scarlet Letter* as Dialectic of Temperament and Idea. *Studies in the Novel*, *23*(1).

Swann, C. (2007). Past Imperfect, Present Imperfect, Future Perfect? In H. Bloom (Ed.), *Nathaniel Hawthorne's The Scarlet Letter*. New York: Chelsea House.

Tassi, N. (1998). Prisons: Sex, Intellect, and Gender in *The Scarlet Letter*. *CEA Critic*, *60*(3).

Thomas, B. (2004). Love, Politics, Justice in *The Scarlet Letter*. In R. H. Millington (Ed.), *Cambridge Companion to Nathaniel Hawthorne*. Cambridge University Press.

Tomc, S. (2002). A Change of Art: Hester, Hawthorne, and the Service of Love. *Nineteenth-Century Literature*, *56*(4).

Ullén, M. (2004). *The Half-Vanished Structure: Hawthorne's Allegorical Dialectics*. Bern: Peter Lang.

Valenti, P. D. (2014). 'Then, All Was Spoken!' What 'The Custom House' and *The Scarlet Letter* Disclose. *Nathaniel Hawthorne Review*, *40*, 19–39.

Wagenknecht, E. (1989). *Nathaniel Hawthorne: The Man, His Tales and Romances*. New York: Continuum.

Afterword

Hawthorne Beyond the Couch

In these chapters, we have peered into the haunted mind of Hawthorne's protagonists and from that vantage have applied a psychoanalytic narrative technique to bring into interpretive coherence their occult psychological crises and the momentous transformations that arise from them. We have followed the characters through unique narrative gaps to their unanticipated ends: Hester and Dimmesdale, in different ways, find spiritual regeneration; Holgrave finds love and reconciliation; Zenobia, tragically, finds release in death; Miriam, overcoming trauma, opens a loving heart to devotion and sacrifice. These transformations, I think I have shown convincingly, occupy the romances' structural and thematic cores. Psychoanalytic technique has proven uniquely poised to penetrate them. Whether this method can be applied as fruitfully to other authors who present similar interpretive dilemmas will be up to my psychoanalytic and literary colleagues, both present and future, to explore.

It is my hope that the interpretations that I have proffered will be useful to all readers of the romances: students, non-specialists, and scholars. Hawthorne's romances are, by design, far from straightforward and readers can lose their way; the psychoanalytic narratives provide a guidance akin to Ariadne's thread. To that end, I have made substantial effort to express psychoanalytic formulation, which can be arcane and off-putting, in a common, accessible language. Moreover, the interpretations arise from close attention to the progression of the texts, which creates for the reader a shared experience of following Hawthorne's written words with me. We are on the same page, as it were, and together we negotiate the narrative gaps the author has thrown in the way; such a proximity facilitates a receptivity to interpretations which are felt to be both right and inevitable.

In that regard, I have been gratified to hear from nonacademic readers of the previously published chapters that the psychoanalytic narratives indeed do shed meaningful and sympathetic light on Hawthorne's characters' plights and bring clarity to the often obscure turns of the plots. These readers have been deeply moved by the romances and express much admiration for

Hawthorne's compelling writing. Needless to say, there is good reason that for generations and worldwide Nathaniel Hawthorne has achieved a unique and esteemed literary status.

I would like to believe that this volume will also make a contribution to the larger context of American literary and Hawthorne scholarship. A systematic psychological explication of Hawthorne's characters has been missing from the critical literature and this work can help make up the deficiency. In some quarters of the Hawthorne scholarly community, there has been resistance to the interpretations contained in these chapters, as many are discordant with what has become commonly accepted wisdom about Hawthorne's protagonists and their fates; academics may not be as willing as non-specialist readers to take this textual journey with me. Every psychoanalyst is accustomed to resistance and has learned that change, if it occurs at all, is often slow and incremental.

However, I believe that whatever an interpreter's perspective, the truth of the human heart is at the center of Hawthorne's fiction. I look forward to this study serving as a resource to inform other interpretive efforts of the details of Hawthorne's psychological imagination which are, after all, such a large part of his rendering of that truth. We will have to wait to see how diverse interpretative perspectives may accommodate to Dimmesdale as a courageous, not cowardly, man and to Hester's return as a fulfillment, not a thwarting, of the self. What will be the critiques of the ending of *The House of the Seven Gables* when it is appreciated that, in having undone the House's centuries-old curse, Holgrave is a hero and not a sell-out? What shifts will take place in critical views of *The Blithedale Romance* when Zenobia's suicide is reimagined as the noble embrace of a tragic destiny not the attention-grabbing act of a histrionic woman? And what will be the commentary on *The Marble Faun* when Miriam, coming out of the shadows that have long enveloped her, can be understood to be a courageous survivor of childhood sexual trauma? It is intriguing to contemplate what will become of Hawthorne beyond the couch.

I also want to acknowledge the limited scope inscribed by this volume. Its argument does not encompass Hawthorne's non-fiction or biography, nor does it situate his work in the context of the American Renaissance. It does not take note of the literary traditions of which he makes use, nor does it compare his fiction with other authors as it relates to style, theme, aesthetics or literary merit. In light of the current trends in criticism, I am aware that the analyses may touch upon, but do not expand, on the romances' historical, social, or political contexts. It is a brand of psychoanalysis that is decidedly Freudian and is not admixed with even a whiff of Lacan; it does not interact in any significant way that I am aware of with gender or feminist studies. This is just the start of its deficiencies, *Mea maxima culpa*. In the end, I have had only one professional life to lead and it has been, until recently, as a psychoanalyst. However, there is a brighter side to these limitations: David Kuhn, to whom this book is dedicated, once speculated that insights of the type offered in this volume most likely could only have been formulated by someone outside the field of literary studies.

Hawthorne has prepared us for the inevitability of a multiplicity of interpretive modes which may organize separately and then join together to capture, as well as they can, the many-colored splendor of a literary work of art. As an end, and here with a different purpose, I repeat the conclusion of Chapter Five, which quotes Hilda's fancy of a story that she will write when she returns home to America: "Would not this be an admirable idea for a mystic story, or parable, or seven-branched allegory, full of poetry, art, philosophy, and religion! It shall be called 'The Recovery of the Sacred Candlestick'. As each branch is lighted, it shall have a differently colored lustre from the other six; and when all the seven are kindled, their radiance shall combine into the intense white light of Truth!" (Vol. 4, p. 371).

Index

For Product Safety Concerns and Information please contact our EU
representative GPSR@taylorandfrancis.com
Taylor & Francis Verlag GmbH, Kaufingerstraße 24, 80331 München, Germany

www.ingramcontent.com/pod-product-compliance
Ingram Content Group UK Ltd.
Pitfield, Milton Keynes, MK11 3LW, UK
UKHW022354190926
475702UK00015B/2280
* 9 7 8 0 3 6 7 7 5 9 1 0 0 *